HEAL
with
AMINO ACIDS
and Nutrients

A Self Help Guide for Common
Health Problems Using Amino
Acids and Natural Remedies—
What to Use and When

Billie J. Sahley, Ph.D., C.N.C.
Katherine M. Birkner, C.R.N.A., Ph.D., C.N.C.

Pain & Stress Publications®
San Antonio, Texas
January 2014

Copyright © 2014 by Pain & Stress Publications®

Note to Readers

This material is not intended to replace services of a physician, nor is it meant to encourage diagnosis and treatment of illness, disease or other medical problems by the layman. This book should not be regarded as a substitute for professional medical treatment and while every care is taken to ensure the accuracy of the content, the authors and the publisher cannot accept legal responsibility for any problem arising out of experimentation with the methods described. Any application of the recommendations set forth in the following pages is at the reader's discretion and sole risk. If you are under a physician's care for any condition, he or she can advise you as to whether the programs described in this book are suitable for you.

No part of this publication may be reproduced, stored in a retrieval system, or transmitted in any form or by any means, electronic, mechanical, photocopying, recording or otherwise, without the prior written permission of the authors.

This publication has been compiled through research resources at the **Pain & Stress Center**, Helotes, Texas 78023.

9th Edition, January 2014
Printed in U.S.A.

A Pain & Stress Publication®
San Antonio, TX 78229

Additional copies may be ordered from:
Pain & Stress Center
17579 Frank Madla Rd. #1, Helotes, TX 78023-3455
1-800-669-2256

Library of Congress Number 2013921115
ISBN 9781889391403 (978-1-889391-40-3)

Acknowledgments and Dedication

Many people pass through our lives whose influence leaves a positive imprint that we carry with us. We dedicate and acknowledge those gifted people for their support, guidance, and dedication to making this world a better place to live and raise our children.

The authors would like to express special thanks to the people who helped make this book possible:

To a new generation of physicians, therapists and educators who seek to find the natural alternative that frees the addicted from the prison of prescription drugs and gives them God's greatest gift—the freedom to make a choice.

To Robert Michael Benson, M.D. who taught me how to live my impossible dream.

To Julian Whitaker, M.D., one of God's gifted healers and an inspiration to all those who reach out.

To the late Candace Pert, Ph.D., neuroscientist, whose research opened many doors in amino acids and neuropeptides.

To David E. Bresler, Ph.D., our mentor in chronic pain and integral medicine.

To Jeffrey Bland, Ph.D., founder of the Institute of Functional Medicine and our mentor for over 25+ years.

To Doris J. Rapp, M.D., whose wisdom and teachings opened the door to the world of environmental medicine.

To Sherry Rogers, M.D. who introduced us to the world of magnesium chloride.

To Annemarie S. Welch, a special physician and friend who shares her wealth of scientific data constantly.

Linda M. Volpenhein, C.N.C., Laura Boyd, B.A., C.N.C. and Deborah Dutcher, whose tireless hours of assistance helped make this book a reality.

To a little boy named Scooter, now, an angel in heaven.

And to the Lord, for always lighting our paths.

A Special Dedication To

My beloved mother for always being with me to guide me, teach me, and encourage me to climb the mountain.

B.J. Sahley

My father for his interest and belief in alternative medicine and his encouragement to explore and look for answers.

My coauthor, Dr. Sahley for her help, encouragement, and belief in me.

K.M. Birkner

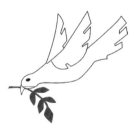

Table of Contents

Introduction 9
Special Information 10
Neurotransmitters, Brain Language 11
    The Synapse 14
Blood-Brain-Barrier 16
    Amino Acids for Brain and Body Function 18
Understanding Amino Acids/Proteins 20
    Proteogenic Amino Acids 20
    Proteins 20
    Classification of Amino Acids 21
Neurotransmitters & Neuropeptides 22
    Limbic System & Mental Distress Pathways 24
Amino Acids and Their Functions 25
    Alanine 25
    Arginine 26
    Asparagine 30
    Aspartic Acid 31
    Branched Chain Amino Acids (BCAA) 32
    Carnitine 36
    Acetyl-L-Carnitine 41
    Cysteine and Cystine 42
    GABA, The Anxiety Amino Acid 45
    Glutamic Acid 48
    Glutamine 49
    Neurotransmitters in Brain Function 53
    Glycine 56
    Histidine 57
    Lysine 58
    Methionine 59
    SAMe (S-Adenosyl Methionine) 61
    Ornithine 63
    Phenylalanine 64
    Proline 66
    Serine 67
    Taurine 68
    Theanine 72
    Threonine 74
    Tryptophan 75
    Tyrosine 79
    S.B.N.C. (Super Balanced Neurotransmitter Complex) ... 80
    Disorders Associated with Amino Acids Imbalances 81
    Amino Acid Cofactors 82
        B6 (Pyridoxine) 83
        U.S. Recommended Daily Allowance for B6 83

  Signs and Symptoms of Vitamin B6 Deficiency 84
  Timed Release Rodex B6 86
  P5'P or Pyridoxal 5' Phosphate (Active B6) 86
  Magnesium 86
    Magnesium/Amino Acid Connection 87
    Drugs that Deplete Magnesium 91
  Alpha KG 89
    Amino Acids and Metabolic Pathways 91
Important Note 92
Amino Acids in Therapy 91
  Acne 93
  Addiction (Alcohol) 92
  Adult A.D.D./Hyperactivity 97
  Allergies/Sinus Problems 100
  Anti-Aging 103
    Decline of Growth Hormone 106
    Brain Boosters (Memory and Concentration) 112
  Carpal Tunnel Syndrome (Repetitive Stress Injury) 119
  Chronic Emotional Fatigue 121
    Symptoms of Chronic Emotional Fatigue and
      Chronic Stress Syndrome 122
  Chronic Pain 128
  Depression 132
    Major Symptoms of Depression 133
    Bipolar (Manic-Depression) 137
      Manic Symptoms 138
  Diabetes 140
  Amino Acids and the Elderly 144
    Ingestion % of Daily Value in People Over 60 144
    Function, Cognition, and Behavior Influenced by Nutrients 145
    Vascular Dementia Symptoms 148
  Grief 150
    Physical Sensations Most Commonly Experienced
      from Grief 151
    Grieving Process 152
    Grief from Pet Loss 154
  Headaches 152
  Heart Disease 162
    Risk Factors for Heart Disease 163
  Hepatitis C 167
  Herpes 170
  Immune Health Support 172
    Vitamin D 173
    Iodine 174
      Iodine Deficiency is a Worldwide Problem 175
    Probiotics 176
  Irritable Bowel Syndrome (IBS) 178
  Insomnia 181
    Causes of Short-Term and Intermittent Insomnia ... 181

Causes of Ongoing Insomnia 182
Leaky Gut Syndrome (LGS) 184
    Causes of LGS 185
    Symptoms Associated with LGS 186
    Common Conditions Associated with LGS 187
Menopausal Stress/Anxiety 189
    Effects of Estrogen Loss 190
    Compounds of Plants with Estrogen-Like Activity . 191
Obsessive-Compulsive Disorder (OCD) 194
Osteoarthritis 197
Panic Disorder 201
    Panic Attack Symptoms 202
Periodontal Disease 205
Premenstrual Syndrome (PMS) 207
    Categories of PMS Symptoms 207
Post Traumatic Stress Disorder (PTSD) 210
    Post-Trauma Case History 214
Seasonal Affective Disorder (SAD) 215
    Direct Circadian Rhythm Influencers 216
    Drugs that Deplete Melatonin 216
Teen Anger and Aggression 218
Low Serotonin Deficiency Symptoms 218
Tourette's Syndrome 222
Amino Acid Testing 227
    Acid Analysis Has Proven Helpful With 227
General Summary of Amino Acids 230
    Alanine 230
    Arginine 230
    Aspartic Acid 231
    Carnitine 231
    Acetyl-L-Carnitine 232
    Citrulline 232
    Cysteine 232
    Cystine 233
    GABA 234
    Glutamic Acid 234
    Glutamine 235
    Glutathione 236
    Glycine 236
    Histidine 236
    Isoleucine 237
    Leucine 238
    Lysine 238
    Methionine 239
    Orthinine 240
    Phenylalanine 240
    Proline 240
    Taurine 241
    Theanine 242

Threonine 243
　　　Tryptophan (5-HTP or 5-hydroxytryptophan) 243
　　　Tyrosine 244
　　　Valine 245
Food Sources of Some Amino Acids 246
Quick Reference 248
　　　Anti-Aging... 249
　　　Aggressiveness.. 249
　　　Alzheimer's Disease.. 249
　　　Arthritis (Osteo) 249
　　　Autism 250
　　　Body Building 250
　　　Cancer 250
　　　Cholesterol 250
　　　Chronic Illness.. 250
　　　Chronic Pain 251
　　　Depression... 251
　　　Diabetes 251
　　　Drug Addiction... 251
　　　Energy 252
　　　Epilepsy... 252
　　　Gallbladder 252
　　　Heart Failure 252
　　　Hepatitis C 252
　　　Hyperactivity 253
　　　Hypertension 253
　　　Hypoglycemia... 253
　　　Insomnia 253
　　　Leg Ulcers 253
　　　Liver Disease 253
　　　Mania 254
　　　Memory/Concentration.. 254
　　　Mental Alertness 254
　　　Parkinson's Disease.. 254
　　　Radiation... 254
　　　Renal Failure 254
　　　Schizophrenia 254
　　　Seizures... 255
　　　Stress 255
　　　Surgery.. 255
　　　Tardive Dyskinesia... 255
　　　Tobacco Addiction... 255
　　　Weight Control... 255
Drug-Nutrient Actions.. 256
Product Information 257
Bibliography 258
Index 277
Other Publications from Pain & Stress Publications® 283
About the Authors 288

Introduction

The late Carl Pfeiffer, M.D., Ph.D., known throughout the world for his work with amino acids and brain chemistry, summarized *orthomolecular therapy* as a means of supplying the brain and cells with the right mixture of nutrients. Dr. Pfeiffer stated, "Many diseases are known to be the wrong balance of essential amino acids and nutrients in the body. Adjusting the diet, eliminating junk foods and ingesting the proper doses of essential vitamins, minerals and amino acids, can correct the chemical imbalance of disease."

The orthomolecular approach helps patients become more aware of our dangerously polluted environment and nutrient-stripped refined foods. The orthomolecular approach is both corrective and preventative. Mega nutrient therapy has become a part of orthomolecular medicine. While it is becoming widely recognized that orthomolecular therapy cures patients by correcting brain chemical imbalances, it is little known that in certain combinations of mega nutrients can be as immediately effective as potent pain-killers or tranquilizers. Mega nutrients treat the whole person's biochemical imbalances; they can be of immediate and long-term benefit. The type of treatment offered by orthomolecular doctors and therapists varies, but the mainstream of work focuses on mega nutrient therapy and diagnostic tests, and treatment with adequate nutrients is a distinguishing characteristic of orthomolecular medicine.

Orthomolecular therapy takes into consideration that every individual is biochemically unique requiring different nutrients and amino acids. With application of this therapy, each individual's need is met, and the mind and body are in a state of homeostasis—a condition where everything in the body is in balance and capable of resisting environmental changes, while regulating internal metabolic function. The difference of how your genes express depends on the nutrients your body has. Simply, nutrients determine your gene expression and control them. In *Orthomolecular Medicine for Physicians* Dr. Hoffer states, "Every tissue of the body is affected by nutrition. Under conditions of poor nutrition, the kidneys stop filtering, the stomach stops digesting, the adrenals stop secreting, and other organs follow suit."

Good nutrition is essential to the preservation of health and the prevention of disease. Mega nutrient therapy has become a part of orthomolecular medicine. It has continually expanded and now recognizes that all of our biological interactions with food, water, air, and light are an important part of good health and prevention of illness, if taken in proper amounts.

Special Information

The major focus of this book is amino acids and nutrients. As you will notice at times we discuss the use of herbs, vitamins, minerals and other important nutrients. We included this important information so that you would be aware of all available options for maximum benefit. All of the products described in this book are used at the Pain & Stress Center in our orthomolecular program.

One of the major functions of the Pain & Stress Center is research. Our goal through research is to supply our readers, patients and customers with the latest information to help you and your family achieve optimum health. *If you have any questions regarding any of the products discussed in this book,* call the Pain & Stress Center at 1-800-669-2256.

You will notice under some conditions such as Depression, we mention several products. *This does not mean you need all of the products. Use the nutrients that fit your symptoms.* You may find some work better for you than others. Everyone is biochemically unique, and responds to supplements in a different way. Our goal is to give you all of the information available to help you find the best and most effective resources for you.

Neurotransmitters, Brain Language

Amino acids and brain function go hand in hand. Understanding your brain function gives you a more comprehensive picture of how to use various amino acids to effectively treat pain, stress, anxiety, and depression. Your body needs and uses basic nutrients every day. These include vitamins, minerals, proteins, carbohydrates, and fats. If you take the water and fat out of your body, 75% of the remainder is protein (amino acids). Muscles, cell membranes, enzymes, and the neurotransmitters are all proteins.

The brain controls every cell in the human body. Its commanding presence is responsible for all sensation, movement, thought, behavior, and a lifetime of memories and dreams. The importance of a healthy, well-nourished, efficiently functioning brain cannot be overstated. This three-pound power pack comprises less than 2% of your total body weight. Your brain regulates your breathing, heartbeat, body temperature, and hormone balance. Speech at any level would be impossible without needed nutrients for proper brain function.

Yet, in spite of the absolute importance of a smoothly functioning brain, it is the most poorly nourished organ in the human body. Ten billion neurons (brain cells) cry to be fed constantly. They need amino acids, vitamins, minerals, oxygen, and fatty acids. The neurons' needs must be satisfied every minute of every day of your entire life. All these nutrients are supplied to the brain via the bloodstream. If blood flow to the brain is interrupted even for 20 seconds, unconsciousness will result. If this mighty power pack is deprived of blood or oxygen for more than 7 to 10 minutes, it will die. The brain feeds on energy in the form of the chemical ATP; adenosine triphosphate. This energy fuels the neurotransmitters, the chemical language of the brain, conducts electrical impulses, transports proteins throughout the cells, extends new nerve connections to other brain cells, and rebuilds worn-out cell membranes. The brain must create its own energy for the billions of neurons that it must feed, and cannot borrow or steal this energy from other parts of the body.

How does the brain make this energy? Inside each neuron resides hundreds of little structures called mitochondria. These function as power plants for the cells. These little power plants burn fuel to generate crucial ATP energy. The brain's very life depends on it. While virtually all organs and tissues of the human body can burn either fat or sugar for fuel, the brain can burn only sugar (glucose) under normal, non fasting conditions. This glucose requirement creates potential problems for the brain. The brain cannot store sugar in its cells, so it totally depends on a second-by-second fuel delivery by the blood circulating through the brain. Brain cells use 50% of all glucose in the bloodstream for fuel and 20% of all inhaled oxygen. The brain's ability to claim this large amount of glucose depends upon a bloodstream relatively free of the blood-sugar lowering hormone, insulin; thus, the importance of chromium picolinate in the diet, as it inhibits the release of insulin.

The way to ensure adequate glucose to the brain is to avoid simple sugar foods such as candy, pastries, drinks, etc. These high-sugar foods easily and powerfully trigger insulin release. Complex carbohydrate foods such as whole grains, vegetables, nuts, peas, beans, and seeds are much more desirable and a brain-friendly source of sugar. They are nature's timed-release sugar supplements.

Each of the brain's billions of neurons functions as a microcomputer. Inside each neuron, nerve impulses are conducted electrically. However, when information exchanges from one neuron to another, the brain uses chemicals called *neurotransmitters* to allow brain cells to communicate with each other (chemical language).

There are approximately fifty different neurotransmitters, but the communication conducted between brain cells uses only about ten major neurotransmitters. Certain neurotransmitters carry pain sensations, while others order voluntary muscle movement; some cause excitatory emotional responses, others are inhibitory. The neurotransmitters that govern our excitatory emotional responses are called catecholamines, noradrenaline (norepinephrine), and adrenaline (epinephrine), that derive from the amino acids phenylalanine and tyrosine. Our reactions to everything we encounter, the way we are stirred by a song or an old picture, angered by an argument or emotional pain inflicted by someone we love, or amused by something we see on television—all depend on the chemical language of the brain; specifically, neurotransmitters. Too much or too little of any of these substances will make us under or overreact according to the stimulus.

How we feed the brain directly affects our production of neurotransmitters. Neurotransmitters determine our mental and emotional state of well-being. Proper nutrition and supplementation can correct or enhance mind, mood, memory, and behavior.

No drug currently in wide use, medical or recreational, addresses the root of neurotransmitter problems. Drugs merely stimulate temporary excessive release of preexisting neurotransmitter stores. They do not increase production of neurotransmitters. This fact explains why drugs often lose their effect over time, with chronic use. Once preexisting neurotransmitter stores are exhausted, the drug is unable to stimulate further neurotransmitter release into the synapses between neurons. Hence, the phenomenon known as drug-abuse "crash" frequently occurs.

Greater transport into the brain of the relevant amino acids, vitamins, and minerals augment nourishment of the brain when there are less-than-adequate neurotransmitter levels. And this, in turn, requires higher levels of amino acids, vitamins, and minerals. If levels of these nutrients in the typical American junk food diet truly and adequately promoted optimal neurotransmitter levels in the brain, we would not be seeing the epidemic level in the U.S. of anti-depressant, anti-anxiety, anti-manic, anti-schizophrenic, and recreational drug use. Virtually all these drugs act either by increasing the synaptic release of brain cell neurotransmitters, without increasing their production, or by pinch-hitting for neurotransmitters whose synaptic levels are chronically low.

All substances of abuse either raise or lower consciousness, and deplete the available neurotransmitters needed to prevent or alleviate depressed moods. When you use drugs escape is the primary goal, but you cannot escape

The Synapse

In the brain, neurotransmitters like serotonin and norepinephrine carry signals from one nerve to the next across the gap (synapse) between the two. Tryptophan enters the pre-synaptic nerve cell, where it converts to serotonin. As more tryptophan enters the cell, more serotonin releases into the synapse. Antidepressant drugs work by keeping more neurotransmitters in the synapse.

stress, anxiety, depression, or grief. You merely prolong the healing process. Prescription drugs for stress do not restore or resolve, they merely use available neurotransmitters.

All major neurotransmitters are made from amino acids and from dietary protein. One of the dangers of a low-protein diet includes not producing enough amino acids to make adequate brain neurotransmitters. Apathy, lethargy, difficulty concentrating, loss of interest, and insomnia all result from not enough amino acids in the diet. ADD and hyperactive children, as well as adults, have low levels of neurotransmitters. Drug use does not produce or increase production of neurotransmitters. Drugs only address symptoms.

Children, as well as adults, who use drugs or alcohol for a long time have dangerously low levels of neurotransmitters. They display panic and anxiety because of the deficiency of neurotransmitters. Once proper supplementation is achieved, the symptoms of panic and anxiety decrease noticeably. You cannot restore the brain chemistry overnight by mega dosing. Deficiencies must be established, then adequate amounts of amino acids, vitamins, and minerals must be implemented. All this is part of the healing process. You have taken the first step by purchasing this book.

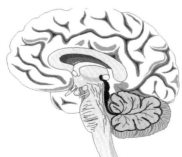

Restore Your Brain . . .

Give your brain the neurotransmitters it needs *daily* to function properly!

Blood-Brain-Barrier
The Protective Barrier

In 1968 Dr. Linus Pauling published an article in *Science* magazine describing the unique function of the "blood-brain-barrier." Dr. Pauling postulated the brain's disadvantage in acquiring the high levels of vitamins and minerals it needs is due to the presence in the brain of a unique blood-brain-barrier (BBB). The BBBs major purpose is to protect the brain from water-soluble toxins. Ironically, however, most of the major brain nutrients—glucose, Vitamins B and C, minerals, and amino acids—are all water soluble. Therefore, the BBB makes it difficult for the brain to absorb the large nutrients needed for delivery to other organs and tissues.

Scientific studies reported by the National Institute of Health (NIH) reveal mild nutrient deficiencies typically cause changes in mood and behavior. Other memory and mental abnormalities will present early detectable signs of nutrient deficiency. Dr. Pauling recommended an increase in the daily intake of B6, Vitamin C, and magnesium. This is far beyond the Percent of Daily Value (% of Daily Value) levels as this produces higher blood levels of these nutrients, thus increasing their penetration of the blood-brain-barrier.

Research done at M.I.T. as early as 1970 pointed to a conclusion that brain neurotransmitter levels were controlled totally by the brain, itself, independent of dietary intake of various amino acids. Further research at M.I.T. pointed to brain neurotransmitter levels are significantly influenced by a single meal. A meal rich in protein will encourage high adrenaline/norepinephrine levels with consequent high alertness and assertiveness. A meal rich in simple sugars and low in protein usually increases brain serotonin levels. This leads to a very relaxed or even, sleepy state.

Alan Gelenberg, M.D., Department of Psychiatry at Harvard Medical School, found tyrosine to be more effective than antidepressants. Dr. Gelenberg noted that those with stress burnout and overload responded extremely well to tyrosine and B6. Tyrosine is the amino acid precursor of noradrenaline, adrenaline, and dopamine.

Glutamine, one of the most plentiful amino acids in the brain, provides a major alternative fuel source for the brain with low blood sugar levels. The amino acid, glycine, also helps alleviate sugar cravings, or that low feeling in the mid-afternoon. Glutamine is important as the precursor for GABA (Gamma Amino Butyric Acid). GABA and glutamine help with problems of concentration and A.D.D. Glutamine also helps the brain dispose of waste ammonia, a protein breakdown by-product irritating to the brain cells even at low levels.

Adequate vitamin and mineral intake also promotes optimum brain neurotransmitter production. B6 is essential to convert all amino acids. Pyridoxal 5' Phosphate (P5'P), the active or coenzyme form of Vitamin B6, is essential to carbohydrate, fat, and especially, protein metabolism. P5'P can be used in place of B6, and is safe for children, and has no adverse side effects. The importance in providing optimal brain nutrition to facilitate optimal brain neurotransmitter production cannot be overemphasized.

Neurotransmitters are produced within neurons and stored in small packets, called vesicles, near the end of the neurons. People are unaware of their brain's activity. The limbic system, the feelings part of the brain, stores all fears of the past, present, and future. The GABA receptor sites control the firing of anxiety-related messages at the cortex, the decision-making part of the brain. The brain's power plant never shuts down and must be fed constantly. When an electrical current

Amino Acids for Brain and Body Function

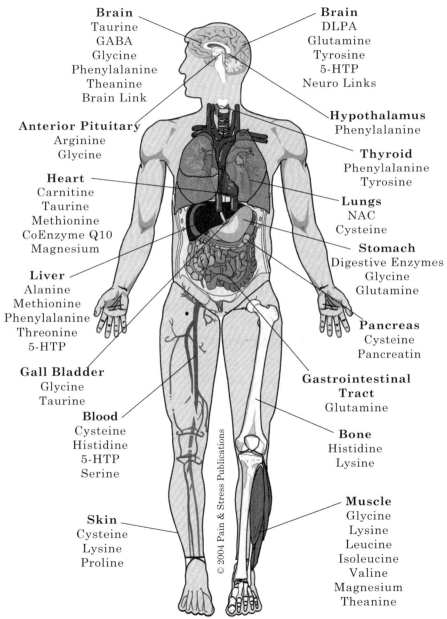

Always add magnesium and B6 or P5'P to all amino acids.

flashes down the length of a neuron, neurotransmitter molecules secrete into microscopic synaptic gaps between two adjacent neurons. Once secreted into the synaptic gap, or synapse between two neurons, the enzymes in the synapse either destroy the neurotransmitters' molecules, or recycle back into the preceding neuron.

> *Neurotransmitters* are the brain's link to smooth brain function.

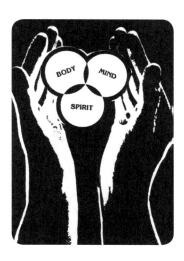

Understanding Amino Acids and Proteins

Proteins control almost every biochemical reaction in the body. All proteins derive from amino acids and are commonly called the *building blocks of life*. If you remove the water and fat from the body, amino acids comprise

Proteogenic Amino Acids

Nonessential	Essential
Alanine	Histidine
Aspartic Acid	Lysine
Arginine	Methionine
Asparagine	Phenylalanine
Cysteine	Threonine
GABA	Tryptophan
Glutamic Acid	Valine
Glutamine	Isoleucine
Proline	Leucine
Serine	
Tyrosine	

Proteins
Six Functional Proteins Divisions

Function	Example
Regulatory proteins	Hormones
Immune proteins	Immunoglobulins
Transport proteins	Hemoglobin
Contractile proteins	Muscle tissue
Structural proteins	Collagen
Enzymes	Proteinase

Source: *Interpretation Guide To Amino Acid Metabolism and Analysis*, Aatron Medical Services

75% of what remains.

All the nearly 40,000 distinct proteins found in the human body are made from only 20 amino acids called the proteogenic amino acids. Amino acids can be broken down into essential and nonessential categories. The body cannot synthesize essential amino acids; they *must* be obtained from the diet. Nonessentials can be synthesized in the body, and are not mandatory in the diet. Although the body can manufacture nonessential amino acids, an abnormality or error in the production of the nonessential amino acids can be metabolically detrimental. Some become conditionally essential amino acids under certain circumstances; i.e., infancy, illness, stress, etc.

Most of the protein in the body resides in the skeletal muscles. Only 0.1% of all protein is found as free amino acids. Plasma amino acids represent what is available to the body at the current time. A deficiency in one of the proteogenic amino acids can limit the body's ability to make an optimal number of certain proteins. Deficiency of amino acids result in both health and disease.

Classification of Amino Acids

Nonessential	*Conditionally Essential*	*Essential*
Alanine	Arginine	Histidine
Asparagine	Cysteine	Isoleucine
Aspartic Acid	Cystine	Leucine
Carnitine	Glutamine	Lysine
Glutamic Acid	Taurine	Methionine
Glycine	Tyrosine	Phenylalanine
Proline		Theanine
Serine		Threonine
		Tryptophan
		Valine

Neurotransmitters & Neuropeptides

The late Dr. Candace Pert was Scientific Director of Rapid Pharmaceuticals. She was a research professor of Department of Physiology and Biophysics at George Washington University School of Medicine. She served as Chief of the Brain Biochemistry and Clinical Neuroscience section at National Institute of Mental Health. Dr. Pert discovered the opiate, GABA, and many other peptide receptors in the brain and body. Her discoveries led to an understanding of the chemicals that travel between the mind and body, such as neurotransmitters.

Everything in your body is being run by messenger molecules called neuropeptides or neurotransmitters. A peptide is made up of amino acids, the building blocks of proteins. Peptides are amino acids strung together very much like pearls strung in a necklace. Peptides are found throughout the brain and body. They are extremely important because they mediate intercellular communication throughout the brain and body. Dr. Pert called neuropeptides and their receptors "the biochemical correlates of emotion."

Within the brain itself are about sixty neuropeptides. Peptides are found in the parts of the brain that mediate emotion. Neuropeptides allow the systems of the body to talk to each other. They control the opening and closing of the blood vessels in your face and throughout the body. Neuropeptides carry messages within the brain, and from the brain to all the body. Neuropeptides direct energy in the body to where it is needed the most. During times of high stress, energy must be directed not only to the brain, but to those parts of the body directly affected by the stress.

One reason the amino acid, GABA, so effectively relieves stress and anxiety is because it is able to reach the GABA receptors throughout the body and brain. Dr. Pert's research established two realms of emotion—physical and mental, found in every cell of your body. In her book, *Molecules of Emotion*, Dr. Pert stated "Emotions are at the nexus between matter and mind, going back and forth between the two and influencing both." The molecular basis of our emotions is inseparable from our physiology. Part of being a healthy person means being well integrated and at peace, with all systems acting together. Neuropeptides and neurotransmitters are the keys to understanding our fear, anxiety, depression, and every emotion we feel.

The study of GABA, other amino acids, and how they affect the brain and behavior is making substantial contributions to the understanding of disease in man. Research done in the field of psychoneuroimmunology confirms disease can originate from within individuals. Major contributing factors include continuous stress overload, the environment, nutrient imbalances, and changes in brain chemistry. The immune system directly effects stress and the quality of life. The different functions of amino acids and how they affect the brain and behavior provide a major focal project for scientists and researchers.

A new age of medicine has emerged, and incorporates the substantial evidence that nutrient deficiencies can and do influence mind, mood, memory, and behavior. Amino acid requirements in the body and brain are tremendously increased by disease and inborn metabolic errors. Any time a person undergoes prolonged periods of stress, anxiety, depression, or grief, they require more amino acids; some more than others. The reason for the different requirements: biochemical individuality.

Every individual has a distinct chemical composition. The brain, glands, and bones are distinct for each person, not only in anatomy, but also in chemical composition. This does not mean that chemical compositions are fixed throughout life, or that they are not influenced by nutrition. Nutrition and amino acid deficiencies affect every tissue in the body, and most importantly, the brain.

Limbic System & Mental Distress Pathways

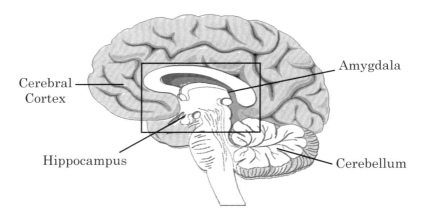

The limbic system is the region of the brain where emotion and moods are regulated and conveyed to the cerebral cortex. The limbic system contains the inhibitory neurotransmitters, GABA, glutamine, glycine, and serotonin that modulate anxiety messages in the brain. The limbic system functions as a crossover zone where signals are transmitted from the rest of the cortex into the limbic system. The limbic cortex is a link to the cerebral cortex for the control of behavior. The complex and powerful amygdala, as part of the limbic system, is the storehouse of memories, emotions, and especially traumatic experiences. Research documents the amygdala as probably functioning at birth; this accounts for negative experiences of our inner child that remain in the amygdala as unresolved anxiety, anger, and fear.

Amino Acids and Their Functions

Alanine

Alanine is a non-essential amino acid and is synthesized in the body. Alanine functions as an inhibitory neurotransmitter in the brain. Highest concentrations of alanine are found in the muscles. During hypoglycemia or in times of need, alanine provides an alternative source of glucose from the liver. Alanine is also present in the prostate fluid and may perform a function in prostate health. A study of 45 men with BPH (benign prostatic hypertrophy) established that 780 mg of alanine per day for two weeks and then a reduced amount of 390 mg for another two and one-half months along with equal amounts of glycine and glutamine reduced BPH symptoms.

Elevated alanine levels in the blood can cause drug-resistant seizure disorders or severe depression. Low alanine levels are often seen with low glycine and taurine, and when the Branched Chain Amino Acids (BCAAs) are deficient. Normal alanine metabolism requires the presence of B6. Alanine is essential for the normal metabolism of tryptophan.

Best food sources for alanine include yeast, spirulina, seaweed (kelp), sesame seeds, soy, fish, beef, gelatins, wheat germ, turkey, duck, cottage cheese, and sausage. Usual supplemental dose range is 200 to 800 mg, daily.

Arginine

Arginine, an essential amino acid, participates in many vital biochemical reactions in the brain and body, and is secreted by the anterior pituitary gland. Arginine is found in proteins consumed in the average diet, and can either be metabolized for glucose synthesis or catabolized to produce energy. Arginine performs specific and vital tasks in the body. Arginine builds muscle, enhances fat metabolism, assists in the release of growth hormone from the pituitary gland, increases sperm count and mobility in some individuals, and fights off infections.

Arginine normally constitutes approximately 5 to 7% of the amino acid content of a normal, healthy adult diet. Arginine transports via the gastrointestinal tract, and absorption occurs in the small intestine. Creatine, the high-energy supplement, forms from arginine. Creatine is used for muscle contraction, strength, and energy. Arginine is important in muscle metabolism because it provides a vehicle for transport, storage, and excretion of nitrogen. Subnormal levels of arginine are consistent with muscle weakness, fatigue, and chronic infections.

Recently, researchers found that arginine prevents clotting without increasing the risk of hemorrhagic stroke, ulcers, gastric bleeding, or kidney damage that is seen with aspirin and other anti-coagulants. In 1994 researchers at Hanover Medical School in Germany gave arginine intravenously. Platelet aggregation (clumping) decreased by 33%. Too much aggregation in blood vessels increases the risk of heart attacks. Dr. Radomski discovered that the blood platelets contain an enzyme called nitric oxide synthase. This enzyme is used to make nitric oxide (NO) from arginine. Endothelial (endothelium) cells line the inside of blood vessels and they also produce NO. This NO relaxes or vasodilates the blood vessels that facilitates blood flow. Researchers at Stanford University School of Medicine report that L-arginine supplementation is very effective in reversing endothelial dysfunction. If arginine is given orally or intravenously, it prevents or reverses atherosclerosis, increases coronary blood flow in heart disease patients, alleviates intermittent claudication, and improves functional status in heart failure patients. Dosage of L-arginine for heart disease is 5000 mg, twice daily according to Mark Houston, M.D., Clinical Professor of Medicine, Vanderbilt University School of Medicine, and Medical Director at Vascular Institute in Nashville, Tennessee.

In recent years research demonstrates arginine as very beneficial to both men and women for sexual enhancement. As the primary source of nitrogen in the body, arginine is essential to production of the important biomolecule, nitric oxide (NO). Nitric oxide is present in all cells of the body. Nitric oxide forms from arginine and is a vital factor in a number of important homeostatic processes. Research indicates that nitric oxide works with arginine, and plays the major role in a man's ability to have an erection. When sexual stimulation is present, the penile nerves transmit their signals, activating the enzyme that converts arginine into nitric oxide within the penis. The release of nitric oxide triggers the erection process. Viagra cannot produce this nitric oxide.

Scientists believe that the majority of male-impotence cases are caused by poor blood flow through the patient's penis. Insufficient production of nitric oxide in the penis in males and in the vagina in females appears to be the major problem. Arginine goes beyond Viagra's capability naturally; studies at New York School of Medicine support this data.

In the best-selling book *Grow Young with HGH*, Dr. Ronald Klatz reports that Doctors A.W. Zorgniotti and E. F. Lizza gave fifteen patients 2,800 milligrams of arginine, daily, for two weeks. All had renewed sexual performance. Women who used arginine reported improved sexual responsiveness. Researchers believe arginine is effective because it is the precursor of nitric oxide. For a man, nitric oxide performs a key role in initiating and maintaining an erection. Women report increased blood flow in the vaginal area, and they test higher in production of nitric oxide.

Arginine also functions as a neurotransmitter that plays a part in learning and memory. In one study of 16 elderly patients with cardiovascular disease who lived in a nursing home received 1.6 grams of arginine per day for 3 months. A revised form of Hasegawa's Demential scale determined the cognitive function. A score of 30 is perfect and less than 20 reflects dementia. The average score was 16 at the start and 23 at the end of the study. No side effects were noted. The scores had fallen back to 17 three months after discontinuing the arginine. The NO produced from the arginine acted as not only a neurotransmitter, but also a vasodilator that enhanced blood flow to the brain. Aging causes a decrease in nitric oxide levels that may play a role in age related mental decline.

Another study with interstitial cystitis patients showed some promise using 500 mg three times a day (1,500 mg). The arginine group (22%) reported a decrease in pain and a trend toward less urgency while 12% of those in the placebo group improved. NO promotes relaxation of urinary tract smooth muscle and may be a factor by enhancing the immune system and interstitial cystitis. Another study supplemented with either 3 or 10 grams per day of arginine. The active treatment group had a higher dropout rate than the placebo group suggesting that arginine may increase symptoms.

Arginine converts two distinct ways in the body, becoming either nitric oxide or L-ornithine. In regards to cancer, Arginine has two dissimilar actions. If arginine converts to nitric oxide, it helps specific immune cells attack cancer. But the tumor has to be the type that forms antigens that provoke the production of anti-tumor antibodies. If Arginine converts to L-ornithine, it can *promote* cancer growth.

Additionally, most cancer patients have surgery at some point in their treatment, and post operative immune suppression is well acknowledged. In 1992 Pennsylvania researchers reported Arginine has a beneficial effect on the immunity of cancer patients. Patients that had upper gastrointestinal malignancy surgery would only recover key parts of their immunity if given arginine, RNA, and omega 3 fish oils. If not, particular immune responses would remain depressed. Researchers concluded that the three supplements "significantly improved immunologic, metabolic, and clinical outcomes in patients with upper gastrointestinal malignancies undergoing major elective surgery." Another study of patients with colorectal cancer, 30 grams of L-arginine daily for three days prior to surgery caused the tumors to have more antigens for immune cells to zone in on. In a study done at the University of Aberdeen, women with breast cancer who were receiving chemotherapy benefited from Arginine. The women who received 30 grams of Arginine daily for three days before each chemo treatment had better immune response.

In the immune system, nitric oxide protects the body against invading bacteria and parasites. In the brain, where nitric oxide forms in the nerve cells, it spreads in multiple directions and activates all cells in the vicinity. This activation of cells modulates multiple functions, including behavior and gastrointestinal transit flow.

Nitric oxide proves vitally essential for motor learning, coordination, and long-term memory in brain function. Timothy Maher, Ph.D., reports in his continuing education module, that angina pectoris (chest pain), atherosclerosis (hardening of the arteries), coronary artery disease, hypercholesterolemia (excessive cholesterol in the blood), hypertension, and nephrosclerosis (renal stenosis or hardening) associated with diabetes mellitus, all respond to arginine therapy.

Arginine is a very safe and effective amino acid with few side effects. However, if you have a problem with herpes (either type), take one gram of lysine daily for a week before you start taking arginine. This is necessary because arginine provides materials available for herpes replication and will cause an outbreak. Lysine blocks the replication and prevents outbreaks. If you are using arginine on an infant, are pregnant or lactating, elderly, have renal (kidney) function impairment, or have hepatic (liver) function impairment, consult a healthcare practitioner and exercise caution. *Schizophrenics should use arginine with caution. Do not use arginine if you have an active malignancy, severe infection, or diabetic retinopathy.*

Arginine deficiency is associated with rash, hair loss and breakage, poor wound healing, constipation, fatty liver, hepatic cirrhosis, coma, and hypoglycemia. Arginine, as with other amino acids, should always be taken away from mealtimes. Otherwise, amino acids compete for absorption. With proteins present in the foods, allow at least one hour before or after meals. Arginine can be combined with glutamine, ornithine, and lysine to enhance growth-hormone production.

Good food sources include carob, chocolate, cabbage, cottage cheese, cheese, gelatin, soy, yogurt, meats, eggs, brown rice, whole grains, nuts, seeds, popcorn, and raisins.

Asparagine

Asparagine is a non-essential amino acid found mostly in animal proteins. If dietary intake is inadequate, the body makes asparagine from aspartic acid and ATP. Asparagine plays a role in the CNS (central nervous system) for proper functioning and biochemical balance in the brain. Asparagine plays a role in the urea cycle, peptide hormone production, and is used to modulate acute lymphoblastic leukemia.

In 1984 Dr. T. Honda found elevated levels of asparagine in patients after tonic-clonic seizures and infantile spasms. Elevated levels were found in some schizophrenia patients.

Food sources of asparagine include asparagus, dairy products, beef, eggs, and poultry.

Aspartic Acid

Aspartic acid is a non-essential amino acid and a major excitatory neurotransmitter. Formed in the body from glutamic acid with the presence of B6, aspartic acid plays a major role in the metabolism of ammonia and other toxins from the body via the urea cycle. Aspartic acid also metabolizes carbohydrates via the Krebs cycle, and forms constituents of DNA called pyrimidine and orotates. Asparagine forms from ATP and aspartic acid, and can convert back into aspartic acid, if needed by the body. Cellular energy depends directly on aspartic acid. Research indicates aspartic acid may be a stimulator of the thymus gland and the immune system. Irregularities of certain neurotransmitters in the brain such as serotonin may be due to low levels of aspartic acid. The absorption of minerals across the intestinal linings into the blood and into cells requires aspartic acid. Elevated aspartic acid levels may be seen in some patients with depression, epilepsy, stroke, high BCAAs, and low ornithine.

Good food sources of aspartic acid include seaweed (kelp), sesame seeds, soy, meats such as pork, turkey, sausage, chicken, eggs, fish, gelatins, wheat germ, cottage and ricotta cheeses.

Branched Chain Amino Acids
(BCAAs) Leucine, Isoleucine, and Valine

The branched chain amino acids include leucine, isoleucine, and valine. As essential amino acids, BCAAs must be obtained from foods. They are especially involved in stress reactions, energy, and muscle metabolism. BCAAs are unique because the skeletal muscles use them directly as an energy source, and they promote protein synthesis.

The BCAAs are similar structurally, but have different metabolic routes. Leucine solely goes to fats; valine solely to carbohydrates; and isoleucine to both. A valine deficiency appears as neurological defects in the brain. Muscle tremors mark an isoleucine deficiency. Stress states, such as infections, trauma, surgery, fever, cirrhosis, and starvation, require proportionally more leucine than valine or isoleucine. Diseases such as hepatitis, cirrhosis, hepatic coma, chronic renal failure, or liver disease, lower the levels of BCAAs. BCAAs, as well as other amino acids, are commonly fed intravenously to chronically ill patients. The BCAAs, particularly leucine, stimulate protein synthesis, increase the re-utilization of other amino acids in many organs, and decrease protein breakdown.

Isoleucine is involved in blood sugar regulation, muscle development and repair, energy regulation, and hemoglobin development. Isoleucine needs increase after surgery, trauma, sepsis, and for diabetic regulation. Isoleucine acts as a source of energy during strenuous activity and enhances endurance. Aerobic, nonaerobic, strength training, and other hard physical exercise necessitate more isoleucine and other proteins. Chronic renal failure patients have severe deficiencies of isoleucine. Signs of low isoleucine are dizziness, headaches, fatigue, depression, confusion, and irritability. Isoleucine must be acquired from food and cannot be synthesized in the body. Food sources of isoleucine include soy, tofu, seaweed (kelp), spirulina, bakers' yeast, fish, beef, pork, turkey, game meat, chicken and turkey, eggs and egg whites, milk, cottage and parmesan cheese, watercress, horseradish, raw Chinese cabbage, kidney beans, lentils, most seeds, chickpeas, romaine and butter head lettuce, spinach, cashews, and almonds.

Leucine is found abundantly in the muscles and plays a role in its repair. Like isoleucine, leucine is involved in energy regulation. After surgery, traumas, sepsis, wound and diabetic regulation, increased need of leucine occurs due to its nitrogen sparing effects. Leucine stimulates insulin production and blood sugar regulation. Wound healing requires leucine. Parkinson's patients have shown improvement from supplemental leucine. Deficiencies of leucine are rare, but vegans and kidney or liver disease patients are at highest risk for a deficiency. The best food sources of leucine are soy, tofu, seaweed (kelp), spirulina, bakers' yeast, fish, meat—beef, pork, turkey, game meat, chicken and turkey, eggs and egg whites, milk, cottage and regular cheese, seeds, and almonds.

Valine is an essential amino acids that is found abundantly in the muscles. Valine is vital for muscle health—metabolism, muscle tissue repairs, and nitrogen balance. Valine may serve as a source of energy for the muscles. Athletes and body builders use valine as part of the BCAAs to enhance performance. Alcoholics and drug addicts often have major deficiencies of valine, and benefit with supplementation to correct and reverse hepatic encephalopathy (brain damage due to alcohol ingestion) and other degenerative neurological disorders. Trauma and burn patients need valine and other BCAAs for tissue repairs. Deficiencies as a whole are scarce in the U.S. since the American diet is heavy in proteins. Although rare, an acute symptom of too much valine is a crawling sensation on the skin. Overdoses of valine symptoms include delusion, fantasy ideas, and vertigo (dizziness). Food sources of valine are soy, tofu, seaweed (kelp), spirulina, fish, beef, pork, turkey, game meat, chicken and turkey, eggs and egg whites, milk and yogurt, cottage and low fat cheeses, mushrooms, baker's yeast, turnip greens, peas, kidney beans, spinach, broccoli, and seeds.

As stress rises, total caloric intake needs increase, primarily due to increased protein requirements. Stress causes proteins to break down rapidly, and increases amino acid utilization three to four fold. About 30% of the diet should be protein or amino acids, especially when the body undergoes severe stress. But when taken in supplement form, BCAAs decrease the rate of amino acid and protein breakdown. More BCAAs and B6, or P5'P (Pyridoxal 5' Phosphate), are needed as stress or disease accelerates.

Use of the BCAAs by athletes, especially weight lifters, increases available energy. BCAA helps replace steroids used by those who want to build muscle mass. The BCAAs, especially leucine, greatly produce energy under many kinds of stress—from trauma, surgery, fever, infection, muscle training, and weight lifting, and for all kinds of athletic training. With prolonged exercise, about 5 to 10% of the energy used comes from amino acids, especially BCAAs. BCAAs should be used in all stress situations. The amount needed will depend on your physical state and stress level. Normal dosage of BCAAs is 1,000 to 3,000 mg per day, divided. BCAAs should be taken together and not singularly. The ingestion of only one BCAA, particularly leucine, decreases the plasma tissue levels of valine and isoleucine.

Athletes can use BCAAs to prevent muscle breakdown. The liver does not break down the BCAAs easily, so they circulate in the body, competing for absorption against other amino acids, especially tryptophan.

Brain serotonin increases with exercise, as does the ratio of BCAAs to tryptophan. Tryptophan contributes to exercise-induced fatigue, but by increasing your BCAAs during exercise, you postpone this fatigue.

At Stockholm University, during competition, researchers gave six female athletes 7.5 grams of BCAAs in a 6% carbohydrate drink. The researchers report the BCAAs increased the BCAA-to-tryptophan ratio which decreased the athletes' fatigue and increased their mental performance and focus. In another study, these researchers gave the BCAA mixture to seven cyclists. The cyclists experienced a 7% drop in their perceived exertion output and a 15% reduction in mental fatigue. The researchers concluded that the BCAAs improved athletic performance, enabled the athletes to remain more focused, reduced fatigue, and allowed more strenuous exercise.

In another study, done at Karolinska Institute in Stockholm, researchers found similar results in cross-country athletes. The researchers found comparable results to the Stockholm University study—the BCAAs serve as a source of local energy to decrease the breakdown of muscles during endurance exercises. If the BCAAs are available during exercise, they prevent the breakdown of muscle tissues while increasing protein synthesis.

BCAAs have other positive effects on the body. If you are on a reduced-calorie diet, BCAAs help you lose more weight, including more abdominal fat without altering your exercise performance. Inside the muscle cells, the BCAAs help sustain higher testosterone levels. The dosage for BCAAs for increased athletic performance ranges from 6 to 18 grams daily, divided.

Carnitine

Carnitine was discovered in 1905 from extracts of meats, but no physiological role for carnitine could be found until fifty years later. Early research indicated carnitine to be essential to the diet, but later research discovered the body produced carnitine from lysine and methionine, provided sufficient amounts of niacin, Vitamins B6, C, and iron were present. If a carnitine deficiency exists, deficiencies of lysine and methionine also exist. Carnitine levels in the body depend on the kidney function to maintain the proper levels that are lost through urination. If the body is low in carnitine, re-absorption of carnitine becomes more efficient as the kidneys excrete less carnitine. In most cases in the body carnitine acts to reduce oxidative stress.

Carnitine is a non-essential amino acid synthesized from lysine and methionine in the liver, kidney, and brain. Concentrations of carnitine are forty times greater in the muscles than in the plasma. Major sources of carnitine in the diet are meat, especially organ meats such as the liver, fish, and dairy products. Vegetables, grains, and fruits contain little or no carnitine. Vegetarians are therefore more susceptible to not only deficiencies of carnitine, but also of lysine and methionine. Carnitine does not readily cross the blood-brain-barrier.

In 1973 research showed carnitine deficiencies exist in some people for various reasons. Between 1980 and 1983, almost 300 studies were published investigating carnitine's nutritional value and anomalies of carnitine metabolism causing clinical symptoms. Some carnitine deficiency symptoms include impaired lipid (fat) metabolism; lipid accumulation in the skeletal muscles, heart muscle, and liver; and progressive muscle weakness with a buildup of fats in the muscle cells. In children carnitine deficiency may manifest as loss of muscle tone, failure to thrive, swelling in the brain, recurrent infections, hypoglycemia, and heart disturbances.

Carnitine is essential to the transportation of long-chain fatty acids into the cells where the fats can be converted to energy. Recent research indicates carnitine plays an important role in converting stored body fat into energy, energizing the heart, reducing angina attacks, controlling hypoglycemia, and is beneficial with diabetes, liver disease, and kidney disease. Carnitine primarily regulates fat burning in the body. Carnitine transports large fat molecules into the part of the cells where fats can be converted into energy. If your level of Vitamin C is low, you can have an apparent deficiency of carnitine. If carnitine is absent or deficient, many fats cannot be burned. The fats build up within the cell and bloodstream as triglycerides and cholesterol. Carnitine supplementation significantly reduces serum triglycerides and cholesterol levels, while increasing HDL (high density lipids or good cholesterol). Dosages are 1,000 to 3,000 mg per day, divided.

Normal cardiac function is dependent on adequate amounts of carnitine. In angina, carnitine improves oxygen utilization and energy metabolism by the heart muscle. By improving the fat utilization and energy production, carnitine prevents the buildup of toxic fatty acid metabolites. These metabolites can cause cell-membrane damage throughout the heart, contributing to impaired heart-muscle contraction, arrhythmias (irregular beats), and death of the heart muscle. Carnitine supplementation helps prevent the production of these fatty acid metabolites.

Many clinical trials have shown that carnitine improves angina and heart disease, and is beneficial in recovery from a heart attack, arrhythmias, and congestive heart failure. Oral supplementation with carnitine helps normalize heart carnitine levels, thereby allowing the heart to use its limited oxygen supply more efficiently. In one study, patients released from the hospital received 4 grams of carnitine daily, and recovered more quickly from their heart attacks. They showed dramatic improvements in heart rate, blood pressure, rhythm disturbances, angina attacks, and clinical signs of impaired heart function compared to the control group.

Carnitine increases heart rate, pressure rate, heart-pacing duration, and decreases left ventricular and diastolic pressures. It increases muscle strength, and is beneficial to heart patients by increasing exercise endurance at doses of 20 to 40 mg/kg (1,400 to 2,800 mg/day). Other studies indicate that carnitine lowers the exercise heart rate, and extends the time of exercise prior to the onset of angina at doses of 40 mg/kg (about 2,800 mg in 150 pound individuals). Carnitine proves very beneficial in congestive heart patients.

Intermittent claudication is intermittent pain in the calf muscle. This is often described as a cramp or tightness causing pain in the calf, much like angina occurs in the heart. Carnitine improves distances walked without pain in intermittent claudication and other peripheral vascular diseases. In one study, 2 grams of carnitine, twice daily, showed a 75% increase in the walking distance after three weeks of supplementation. This results from the improved energy metabolism within the muscle.

In patients with uremia or kidney disease, carnitine may reduce the risk factor for atherosclerosis and coronary heart disease. Carnitine dramatically reduces triglycerides and cholesterol levels, while increasing HDL (good cholesterol) levels. In addition, carnitine reduces muscle cramping and muscle weakness by restoring muscle carnitine levels. Carnitine deficiencies usually exist in hemodialysis patients due to decreased carnitine synthesis.

Diabetics have reduced blood levels of carnitine. Since cardiovascular disease and reduced kidney and liver function are found in diabetics, supplementing with carnitine is encouraged. Reduced levels of carnitine in skeletal muscles are seen in patients with various muscular dystrophies. The muscular weakness experienced by these patients is believed to result from the low carnitine levels. Carnitine supplementation increases muscle strength, while decreasing lipid levels.

In one study failing heart or patients with congestive heart failure (CHF), carnitine levels was compared to controls. The study showed that the concentration of carnitine in the heart muscle was considerably lower in CHF patients and the level of carnitine was directly related to the ejection fraction of the patients' hearts. Ejection fraction measures the amount of blood volume pumped from the heart with every heartbeat. With CHF, the ejection fraction reduces to as little as 10 to 15% in severe cases. The study showed that carnitine deficiency in the heart directly effects heart function. Another study showed that plasma and urinary carnitine levels could act as markers for heart damage and impaired left ventricular function. Long-term administration of carnitine demonstrated beneficial long term survival with CHF patients in dose range of 2 grams per day.

Carnitine also plays an important role in the production of heat in brown fat. The brown fat helps us acclimate to cold temperatures, and is thought to help determine how much of the food eaten is burned for heat, and how much is stored as body fat. During poor weight loss diets, carnitine prevents the accumulation of ketones in the blood stream. Ketosis can be life threatening, if uncontrolled. And ketonic states can cause the loss of potassium, magnesium, and calcium.

In cancer patients receiving chemotherapy, carnitine has been shown to protect the heart during adriamycin chemotherapy. Additionally, carnitine helps alleviate some of the toxicity associated with chemotherapy through its effect on the mitochondrial integrity.

Carnitine improves the symptoms attributed

to anticonvulsant medications such as Valproic acid (Depakote, Depakene) and carbamezepine (Tegretol and Epitol). Carnitine may offer protection against drug toxicity.

Recent studies indicate carnitine may be a factor with depression. Supplementation with 1,000 mg per day, divided, is helpful.

Carnitine supplementation does not need to be limited to people with cardiovascular problems. Effective utilization of fatty acids by the heart and skeletal muscles depends upon ample supplies of carnitine. Supplementation with 1 to 2 grams, two to three times daily, results in significant improvements in cardiovascular function in response to exercise, especially endurance related activities. It may benefit healthy people as well as athletes by helping burn certain amino acids, called BCAAs or branch chain amino acids in the skeletal muscles. During fasting or prolonged strenuous exercise, the BCAAs provide a significant amount of metabolic energy. Ketones result from the incomplete burning of fat, and are extremely toxic to the nervous system and brain. Carnitine helps to significantly lower the ketone levels.

The daily dose of carnitine ranges between 1,000 to 4,000 mg in divided doses. Carnitine is very safe with no significant side effects in most human studies. But use only the L-carnitine form of carnitine. According to the University of Maryland, only use carnitine under the direction of a health care provider if you are taking AZT (for AIDS), Doxorubicin (chemotherapy agent), Isotretinonin (Accutane for acne), and Valproic acid (anticonvulsant). There may be interactions between carnitine and your medication. When carnitine and coenzyme Q10 are combined, they appear to work synergistically.

Acetyl-L-Carnitine

A subcategory of carnitine is the amino acid, Acetyl-L-Carnitine (ALC). The brain absorbs and utilizes most of the ALC. ALC is the most studied of the carnitines. ALC is more expensive than L-Carnitine. Since ALC crosses the blood brain barrier, ALC has a more observable effect on the brain than carnitine. ALC does improve mental clarity and focus along with mild mood elevation. ALC protects the brain against oxidation and degeneration by preventing cell death. ALC helps to stimulate acetylcholine, a key substance necessary for memory and to connect the brain neurons.

Aging causes a loss of neurons in the brain resulting in slower thinking as the number of neuro-connection pathways diminish. The reduction of age-related neuron loss degrades the thinking process pathways, thinking time, and reaction times. ALC facilitates the release and synthesis of acetylcholine and dopamine from neurons. Acetylcholine is an important neurotransmitter. ALC stimulates neuron growth after 5 days by 5.6%. Whereas a new patented carnitine, ALC arginate stimulates the growth of the neurons by 19.5%.

Studies of ALC with Alzheimer's sufferers show improvements in memory compared to a placebo. An Italian study used 2 grams of ALC daily orally for three months to early stage Alzheimer's patients who had not responded to traditional drug treatment such as Aricept or Exelon. Response times improved by 38% with the acetylcholinesterase inhibitor drugs alone and to 50% with the addition of ALC. Response rates were determined by a variety of functional and behavioral parameters. Another double blind, placebo controlled study done at Stanford University concluded, "Acetyl-L-carnitine slows the progression of Alzheimer's disease in younger subjects."

Other anti-aging benefits of ALC include substantial

improvement in age-associated changes in the brain lipid composition, memory, and reversal of age-associated hearing loss, and improvements in eye lens proteins. ALC also improves heart function due to its ability to enhance mitochondrial activity.

Usual dosage of ALC is 1 gram twice daily, but can be increased to 2 grams with dementias.

Cysteine and Cystine

Cysteine is considered conditionally essential, and is one of the sulfur-containing amino acids. Cysteine is present in almost all forms of protein and the average diet consumes 1 gram of L-cysteine per day. High food sources include ricotta and cottage cheese, yogurt, pork, meats, poultry, wheat germ, granola, and oats.

Cystine is a non-essential amino acid and the stable form of cysteine. Cystine is a component of connective and skeletal tissue, digestive enzymes (papain, trypsinogen, and chromotrypsinogen A), insulin, and hair keratin. Conversion of one to the other occurs in the body, as either is needed. Many foods contain adequate amounts of cystine. The highest include eggs, soy, sesame seeds, meats, beans, grains, nuts, dairy products, and whey.

If Vitamin C is not present, cysteine converts to cystine. Research now focuses on the protective role of dietary amino acids. Cysteine builds proteins, such as those in hair, digestive enzymes, skin, fingernails, and also helps destroy harmful chemicals in the body such as acetaldehyde and free radicals produced by smoking and drinking. Alpha keratin is a protein located throughout the body in different structural tissues that contains the highest concentration of cysteine. Cysteine is an alternative energy source. With extended physical stress cysteine often converts to glucose.

Cysteine spares methionine (another important amino acid) and can completely replace dietary methionine if the diet is supplemented by appropriate amounts of folic acid and Vitamin B12. Cysteine resides abundantly in proteins such as keratin in hair (12%) and trypsinogen (10%). Cysteine acts as a detoxifier. Heavy metals such as mercury, lead, and cadmium will tie up or bind to cysteine so it can be removed from the body.

Cysteine may protect heavy drinkers and smokers against acetaldehyde poisoning from chronic alcohol intake or smoking, according to Dr. Herbert Sprince at the V.A. Hospital in Coatesville, Pennsylvania, and Thomas Jefferson University in Philadelphia.

Pearson reports cysteine is effective, "Not only in preventing hangovers, but also in preventing brain and liver damage from alcohol, and in preventing damage such as emphysema and cancer caused by smoking." Cysteine has been found to offer a degree of protection against radiation exposure.

Dr. William Philpott postulated that cysteine is necessary for the utilization of Vitamin B6. His studies suggest, "A majority of chronic degenerative illnesses, whether physical or mental, have a Vitamin B6 utilization disorder. The culprit causing this Vitamin B6 utilization problem seems to be cysteine deficiency." Dr. Philpott recommends patients having the Vitamin B6 utilization problem take 1.5 grams of L-cysteine three times a day for a month, and then reduce it to twice a day. Vitamin C should always be taken with cysteine.

Diabetics should use cysteine with care because it can cause glucose levels to change and may hamper insulin production.

A specialized modified cysteine known as NAC, or N-Acetyl Cysteine, was first produced by Mead Johnson for the treatment of excess mucus. The primary use for NAC is as a mucus-reducing agent. Mucus strands are broken up to decrease viscosity and congestion associated with excess mucus and sinus drainage. Oral supplementation of NAC is used with allergies, bronchitis, chronic sinusitis, asthma, pneumonia, cystic fibrosis, and even the common cold. Supplemental NAC dosage is usually 600 mg, twice to three times daily.

NAC modulates the production of, and is the precursor to, glutathione. In turn, glutathione helps protect the body against natural and man-made oxidants. Glutathione is an antitoxin and a neurotransmitter. Doctors often use NAC to treat acetaminophen (Tylenol) poisoning. NAC reduces the damage to the kidneys and liver that is associated with this overdose. In the U.S. acetaminophen toxicity is the number one cause of acute liver failure. NAC helps detoxify acetaminophen due its powerful antioxidant, glutathione that derives from NAC, and can be given orally or intravenously to save lives for acute acetaminophen (Tylenol) poisoning.

Recent research indicates when NAC is combined with nitroglycerin, it helps improve the symptoms of heart and coronary artery disease. Complications usually seen in heart disease patients such as chest pain and heart attack occur less frequently and patients receive greater benefit when NAC and nitroglycerin are combined than when either is used alone.

NAC supplementation may prove helpful in auto immune disorders such as Sjogren's syndrome. Some research suggests that NAC may prevent cataracts and macular degeneration, and assist cognitive functioning in Alzheimer's patients.

In early 2010 researchers found that NAC offers some protection against the flu and dual protection against the bird flu. It inhibits replication of the virus and mediates the inflammatory mediators in cells infected with H5N1 virus, and may be an answer if the avian flu goes global.

Another study showed that people using 600 mg of NAC twice daily for 6 months, only 25% of them experienced influenza-like symptoms compared to 79% in the placebo group. The researchers concluded that NAC when taken in the winter time appears to provide a significant attenuation of influenza and influenza like episodes, especially in the elderly high risk individuals.

Usual dosage of NAC is 600 to 1800 mg daily, divided.

GABA
The Anxiety Amino Acid

GABA (Gamma Amino Butyric Acid), an inhibitory neurotransmitter, is found throughout the central nervous system (CNS). GABA assumes an ever-enlarging role as a significant influence on pain, stress, anxiety, and depression as well as stress-induced illnesses. By January 1998, there were over 3,000 documents and texts on GABA, describing how it affects anxiety/stress in the brain.

Dr. Eugene Roberts discovered GABA in 1950. Dr. Roberts established that GABA was involved in the conditions of nerve impulses and thought GABA had widespread distribution throughout the brain and body. In the early 1970s, Dr. Candace Pert, a pharmacologist, documented the GABA receptor sites throughout the brain and body. Dr. Pert's research demonstrated the importance of GABA in the stress-anxiety network.

Of all the brain synapses 40 to 50% of the synapses contain GABA. GABA is the most widely distributed neurotransmitter in the brain and plays a vital role in neuronal and behavioral inhibition. GABA is present in a concentration some 200 to 1000 times greater than neurotransmitters such as acetylcholine, norepinephrine, and 5-HTP. The highest concentration of GABA resides in the basal ganglia followed by the hypothalamus, hippocampus, cortex, amygdala, and thalamus.

If you examine a step-by-step process of what happens in the brain when you feel stress and anxiety, you would see how GABA works to slow down messages. Panic, anxiety, or stress-related messages begin to release numerous signals, and concurrently a physiological response begins to take place—the fight-or-flight syndrome.

The unceasing alert signals from the limbic system eventually overwhelm the cortex (the decision-making part of the brain), and the ability of the cortex and the rest of the stress network becomes exhausted. The balance between the limbic system and the rest of the brain to communicate in an orderly manner depends critically on inhibition. GABA inhibits the cells from firing, diminishing the anxiety-related messages from reaching the cortex.

GABA fills certain receptor sites in the brain and body. This slows down and blocks the excitatory levels of the brain cells that are about to receive the anxiety-related, incoming message. When the message is received by the cortex, it does not overwhelm you with anxiety, panic or pain. You are able to maintain control and remain calm. But, if you are under prolonged stress or anxiety, your brain exhausts all the available GABA and other inhibitory neurotransmitters, thus allowing anxiety, fear, panic and pain to attack you from every direction. Your ability to reason diminishes. In a full blown anxiety or panic attack, physical symptoms include excessive sweating, trembling, muscle tension, weakness, loss of control, disorientation, difficulty breathing, constant fear, headaches, diarrhea, depression, and unsteady legs.

Research done at the Pain & Stress Center, in San Antonio, with patients suffering from all types of stress, pain, muscle spasms or anxiety/panic attacks, demonstrated pure GABA, 375 or 750 mg, can mimic the tranquilizing effects of Valium or Librium without the possibility of addiction or fear of being sedated. GABA fills the receptor in the brain and nourishes the brain with what should be there. Pure GABA dissolves in water, and is tasteless and odorless. The calming effect usually occurs within 10 to 12 minutes.

Tranquilizers provide only temporary relief. We have seen many patients on Xanax that still experience anxiety. They have been told it is not addicting—it is! THERE IS NO SUCH THING AS A TRANQUILIZER DEFICIENCY! Nutrient deficiencies can and do change behavior. Human behavior involves the functioning of the whole nervous system, and the nervous system requires amino acids. GABA, glutamine, and glycine proves vital for energy and the smooth running of brain functions.

B6 (pyridoxine) and Mag Link (magnesium chloride) are GABA's most important partners. We have successfully used GABA, glutamine, and glycine with patients to ease anxiety, muscle pain/spasms, and nervous stomachs. GABA 375 or 750 are free form, not combined with anything else. There is a GABA with niacinamide and inositol on the market, but let me caution you—do not mega dose, with this form. If you do, you will have side effects. Side effects include tingling lips and extremities, rapid heart beat, shortness of breath, flushing, nausea, and increased anxiety. If this occurs, drink 16 ounces of water, and eat a couple of soda crackers. If you weigh less than 125 pounds, use GABA 375, or one-half of a GABA 750 capsule.

Special Note: Magnesium is the stress mineral, and is involved in over 300 enzyme reactions in the body. Take magnesium along with B6. The best form for maximum absorption and tolerance is magnesium chloride (Mag Link). Magnesium chloride is the same form of magnesium present in the body.

Glutamic Acid

Glutamic acid is a non-essential amino acid that can be synthesized by the body, or be converted into glutamine and GABA. Glutamic acid or glutamate is thought to be an excitatory neurotransmitter found in the central nervous system. It acts as a brain ammonia detoxifier. Additionally, glutamic acid provides fuel for the brain, and assists with cognitive functioning.

Since glutamic acid can be manufactured from aspartic acid, ornithine, arginine, proline, and alpha-ketoglutarate, no deficiencies of glutamic acid have ever been seen. Elevation of glutamic acid may be present in some schizophrenics, epileptics, and patients with gout. In fact, epileptics generally have an elevation of glutamic and aspartic acids, and have low levels of GABA, taurine, and glycine.

Glutamic acid may serve as a protective mechanism against heart muscle deterioration in heart disease individuals. Glutamic acid plays a role in normal functioning of the prostate. Large concentrations are found in prostate fluid. In one clinical study of 50 men, symptoms of benign prostatic hypertrophy (BPH) improved considerably with the addition of 780 mg of glutamic acid daily for 2 weeks along with equal amounts of alanine and glycine; then followed with 390 mg of glutamic acid along with alanine and glycine daily for another 2½ months.

Supplementing with more than 3 grams of glutamic acid daily may result in intestinal discomfort, GI disturbances, headaches and the onset of specific neurological conditions such as amyotropic lateral sclerosis (ALS or Lou Gehrig's disease), lathyrism, and Alzheimer's disease.

Rich food sources of glutamic acid include seaweed (kelp), sunflower and sesame seeds, soy, crustaceans such as king crab, shrimp, crayfish, yogurt, cottage cheese, turkey, and chicken.

Glutamine

Glutamine, a conditionally essential amino acid, is the third most abundant amino acid in the blood and brain. The body readily synthesizes glutamine. Normally, in the average diet glutamine consumption from foods is five to ten grams daily. The highest concentrations of glutamine are found in the skeletal muscle, brain, liver, and stomach. Skeletal muscles contain about 60% of the total glutamine stores. When metabolic stress occurs glutamine releases into the bloodstream where it is transported to the tissues in need.

Glutamine, an inhibitory neurotransmitter, acts as a precursor for GABA, the antianxiety amino acid. Glutamine crosses the blood-brain-barrier into the brain, where it increases energy and mental alertness. It helps the brain dispose of waste ammonia, a protein breakdown by-product. Ammonia irritates brain cells, even at low levels. Recent scientific research demonstrates glutamine links to the most important functions of the body's vital organs and musculoskeletal system. Glutamine assists the body in muscle development when illness causes muscle wasting—sometimes seen following a high fever, chronic stress, illness, or a traumatic accident. Glutamine provides a major alternative fuel source for the brain with low blood sugar levels.

In 1980 glutamine was reestablished as a conditionally essential amino acid; prior to 1980, glutamine was considered a non-essential amino acid. A conditionally essential amino acid means that under normal circumstances, the body can make (synthesize) adequate quantities of that amino acid; but in times of stress such as fever, illness, trauma, dieting, or chemotherapy, the body cannot make as much as it requires. An additional amount of the amino acid must be taken in nutrient form to prevent a deficiency.

Glutamine's most important function is strengthening the immune system. Glutamine supports the multiplication of selected white cells that strengthen the body's defense system. Glutamine aids other immune cells in killing bacteria, healing wounds, and maintaining and supporting glutathione, as an important antioxidant. Glutamine also supports pancreatic growth.

Scientists at NIH in 1970 found glutamine to be the most important nutrient for the intestinal tract. During times of illness, the body uses more glutamine to help tissue repair in the kidneys, intestines, and liver. The GI tract is the greatest user of glutamine. The small intestine absorbs the highest amount of glutamine in the body, higher than any other organ in the body. For many years glutamine was considered a non-essential amino acid, but research over the past several years brought forth a wave of new, important information to change this view.

Every day researchers conduct more studies on the healing power of amino acids. Glutamine deserves special attention. Studies show glutamine supplementation during cancer treatment increased the effectiveness of many chemotherapy drugs, and increased tumor kill-off. Systemic infections (sepsis) decreased by up to 80% with glutamine supplementation. The mechanisms appear to be increased intestinal integrity and reduced intestinal ulcerations. Glutamine decreased weight loss and increased nitrogen balance. Following radiation, glutamine decreased mortality to the point of ameliorating toxicity. Additionally, glutamine augmented healing of radiated intestines.

Some amino acids help the body resist the effects of the radiation which is becoming a significant pollutant and potentially, a worldwide problem. In cancer patients, glutamine enhances the effectiveness of chemotherapy and radiation treatments, while reducing the toxicity and damage to the body. Dosages vary in amounts, but a rule of thumb is 0.5 grams/kilogram of body weight daily.

For best results, take glutamine prior to treatment and continue throughout therapy. Research has shown glutamine is the second most important fuel for the cells' lining in the colon.

The main nutrient needed for intestinal repair is glutamine. When trauma such as burns, surgery, hemorrhagic shock, or other physical trauma occur, increased intestinal permeability often results. These traumas re-route glutamine away from the intestines into the bloodstream and into tissues that require it. During these traumatic times, glucocorticoid releases causing accelerated protein breakdown. The skeletal muscles provide glutamine for tissue healing and gut integrity, but loss of systemic glutamine is large when this type of trauma happens. As stores of glutamine deplete, wound healing impairs, derangement of normal intestinal microbes occurs that may result in sepsis or multiple organ failure. Bacteria, fungi, and their toxins translocate across the mucosal barrier into the bloodstream.

Leaky gut syndrome is recognized more often today due to the increased use of anti-inflammatory medications such as Motrin, Advil, Ibuprofen, Anaprox, Aleve, Naprosyn, etc. and steroids. Leaky-gut syndrome makes the intestines more permeable and allows substances and foods which do not normally pass into circulation to cross. Food allergies can result, causing more discomfort and pain. But glutamine helps the gut to heal and makes the intestines less permeable. Japanese researchers found glutamine helps stomach ulcers heal. In the book *The Ultimate Nutrient Glutamine*, Judy Shabert reports that Douglas Wilmore, M.D. of Harvard Medical School found glutamine is a key to the metabolism and maintenance of muscle. Glutamine is the primary energy source for the immune system and factors that are enhanced by growth hormone.

Glutamine helps clear the body of waste through the kidneys and liver. For those with impending surgery, glutamine supplements should be considered before, during, and after surgery. New research demonstrates the body's release of amino acids during times of stress includes one-third in the form of glutamine. Further research revealed the muscles synthesize glutamine as they break down in times of heavy stress. When glutamine was taken with balanced amino acids, muscle breakdown (atrophy) was essentially prevented. A recent study shows the need of glutamine supplementation. Sixty patients with multiple traumas were given glutamine containing enteral nutrition for at least five days following their injuries. Dramatic differences occurred between the glutamine-supplemented group versus the control group. The incidence of pneumonia was 17% in the glutamine group while 45% developed pneumonia in the control group. Bacterial infection occurred in 7% of the glutamine group while 42% of the control group; 1 patient in the glutamine group developed sepsis versus 8 patients in the control group. This suggests that glutamine prevents translocation of bacteria from the gut while providing better protection against infections.

During and after strenuous exercise, glutamine needs increase. In fact, the amount of glutamine is less than what the liver normally produces, and glutamine levels can reduce up to 50%. Catabolism or muscle breakdown happens if the body takes glutamine from the muscles for use somewhere else without replenishing it. Besides muscle breakdown, depressed glutamine levels have an impact on the immune system making athletes more vulnerable to allergies and other infectious diseases. Recent studies demonstrate that exertion has a profound effect on glutamine reserves. In one study, seven healthy athletes doing intensive anaerobic exercise (sprint running) showed a 45% drop in plasma glutamine compared to levels prior to exercising. When the same athletes did intensive aerobic exercise (10 days of cross country running), their plasma glutamine decreased 50%. A portion of the runners continued to have low glutamine levels even 6 days after recovering from the cross-country running. This suggests that these athletes needed to increase their intake of glutamine via diet or with supplementation. Low intensity exercise does not seem to deplete glutamine levels or affect the immune system.

Glutamine is an effective growth hormone stimulator according to Vincent Giampapa, M.D. Dr. Giampapa is a Certified Anti-Aging Physician and Clinical Professor at University of Medicine and Dentistry of New Jersey. In the book, *Grow Young with HGH*, Dr. Klatz reported that two grams of glutamine are more potent than one gram of arginine, ornithine, and lysine combined.

Note: Over the past years there has been confusion regarding glutamine, glutamic acid, and glutamate. Glutamine is not glutamic acid, glutamate, MSG, or glutathione. Glutamine, GABA, and glycine are rapidly becoming the most important therapeutic amino acids of the twenty-first century.

Neurotransmitters in Brain Function

The amino acid trio of glutamine, GABA, and glycine, along with Vitamin B6, the cofactor, represent the major inhibitory neurotransmitters in the brain. Glutamine is found in the nerves of the hippocampus—the memory center of the brain, in the cranial nerves, and in many other areas of the brain. These three amino acids work together, and are inhibitory neurotransmitters. Anyone taking amino acids must take Vitamin B6 to metabolize these amino acids.

Glutamine studies reported that intellectually impaired children and adults demonstrated an increase in IQ after taking glutamine in combination with ginkgo and Vitamin B6. Research done by Dr. Roger Williams at the University of Texas, Clayton Foundation, showed children and adults classified ADHD showed a marked improvement when taking glutamine, 250 mg to 1,000 mg, daily. Dosage depends on age and weight. At the Pain & Stress Center we use a Super Balanced Neurotransmitter Complex along with AC (Anxiety Control 24). If needed, extra glutamine powder and ginkgo are added. Results have been excellent. The Super Balanced Neurotransmitter Complex formula assists brain communication and allows the brain cells to talk to each other. Recent discoveries found 50 or 60 neuropeptides in the immune system, as well as in the brain. Each unique neuropeptide has its own receptor. These intercellular neuropeptides and receptors mediate communication among the brain, glands, and immune system. Neuropeptides are peptides made up of amino acids, the building blocks of proteins. Neuropeptides and their receptors form the biochemical correlates of emotion.

GABA and glutamine are found not only in the brain, but in the receptor sites throughout the body. Amino acids can and do change mind, mood, memory, and behavior. A particular herb, Ginkgo Biloba demonstrates excellent results in enhancing concentration. Ginkgo increases blood flow to the head, and improves mental functioning and the ability to focus for longer periods of time. Ginkgo has also been helpful after a stroke by increasing circulation to the brain. In his book *Herbal Tonic Therapies*, Daniel Mowrey, Ph.D. reviews studies using Ginkgo. In one study patients received 120 mg of ginkgo, daily, for twelve weeks. Patients reported a definite improvement in alertness and memory. Ginkgo and glutamine provide an effective combination for those with problems in concentration, memory, and staying on task. Ginkgo promotes an increased nerve transmission rate, and improves synthesis and turnover of brain neurotransmitters.

For those with alcohol cravings, Dr. Roger Williams' pioneering in glutamine research found 3,000 to 4,000 milligrams of glutamine, daily, will stop the craving for alcohol and decrease the craving for sweets. Since pure pharmaceutical glutamine, such as Super Glutamine, is tasteless, and mixes readily with water or any cool liquid, patients find it easy to take. Patients also reported a lift from fatigue, both mental and physical. One alcoholic stopped drinking when glutamine was administered daily. Two years later the patient was still free from the craving for alcohol. He maintained a nutritional support program. Dr. Lorene Rogers, researcher at the University of Texas, Clayton Foundation, reported several cases in which glutamine was successful and placebos ineffective. Glutamine was given to one group of alcoholics and placebos to the other. The group taking at least 3,000 milligrams of glutamine daily were free of alcohol craving.

The brain converts glutamine to energy, and with glutamine the brain's main fuel, it converts the glutamine to GABA, with the help of magnesium. Without continued high energy in the brain, the rest of the mind and body will NOT function properly. The brain requires a huge supply of glucose and oxygen in order to perform properly. This energy supply transports via the bloodstream. Proper circulation ensures the brain has the glutamine (energy) it needs.

Unfortunately, <u>foods are not a good source of glutamine</u>. The foods highest in glutamine include meat, chicken, and eggs, but in the raw form. Cooking or heating inactivates glutamine, so your best source is supplement form.

Glutamine is available in capsule and powder forms. If using powder form, put in cool water or juice. Heat destroys glutamine.

Glycine

Glycine is a non-essential amino acid, and has the simplest structure of all the amino acids resembling glucose (blood sugar) and glycogen (excess sugar converted in the liver for storage). Glycine is sweet to taste, and can be used as a sweetener. It can mask bitterness and saltiness. Pure glycine dissolves readily in water. As the third major inhibitory neurotransmitter in the brain, glycine readily passes the blood-brain-barrier. The body needs glycine for the formation of DNA, collagen, phospholipids, and for the release of energy.

According to Ronald Kotulak in his book, *Inside the Brain*, glycine "helps trigger brain cells to fire electric charges and speed learning." Glycine helps spasticity and seizures, and is involved in behaviors related to convulsions and retinal function. If taken orally, glycine increases the urinary excretion of uric acid, and is possibly a useful adjunct to gout.

Glycine is an essential intermediate in the metabolism of protein, peptides, and bile salts. Liver detoxification compounds, such as glutathione, must have glycine present for formation. Glycine removes heavy metals such as lead from the body, and also decreases the craving for sugar. In many cases, use some glycine to replace sugar on foods such as cereal. Glycine has been shown to calm aggression in both, children and adults. When combined with GABA and glutamine, glycine influences brain function by slowing down anxiety-related messages from the limbic system. Glycine is effective in alcohol withdrawal as it decreases the craving for sugar.

Glycine plays a role in the regulatory pathways for sleep. Studies show that glycine enhances sleep quality and increases deeper stages of sleep. Glycine should not cause grogginess or a morning hangover when you use 2 to 3 grams of glycine about an hour before retiring. Glycine is available as a powder or capsule.

Recently, a paper reported that glycine protects the brain against energetic disturbances resulting from hypoxic (oxygen deprived) conditions. Glycine is utilized as therapy for ischemic stroke, and a study shows it lengthens the lifespan of cortical neurons under oxygen deprived conditions. Glycine may be the amino acid that may offer neurological protection in people with sleep apnea.

Research indicates that glycine can work as an antibiotic, especially against H. pylori bacteria, which is associated with ulcers and stomach cancer.

Food sources include seaweed (kelp) and spirulina, crustaceans, meats such as ostrich, pork, lamb, buffalo, beef, veal, fish, turkey, soy, watercress, wheat germ, sunflower seeds, spinach, egg whites, chicken, turnips, and gelatin,.

As a very nontoxic amino acid, glycine can be used by both children and adults. Usual dosage range is 500 to 3,000 mg, per day, in divided doses.

Histidine

Histidine, one of the essential amino acid, is required in large amounts in infants. Histidine is necessary for the maintenance of myelin sheaths of nerves, and has vasodilating and mild anti-inflammatory properties. The neurotransmitter, histamine, derives from histidine. Histidine promotes large increases in brain histamine content, especially in the hypothalamus.

People with abnormally high amounts of histamine often demonstrate a history of psychiatric problems ranging from mild to severe. People with chronic pain and fibromyalgia demonstrate high histamine levels represented by joint swelling. High histidine and histamine levels are often seen in patients with obsessive-compulsive disorders, depression, and phobias. Low blood histamine levels are found with rheumatoid arthritis and Parkinson's disease.

Best food sources for histidine include pork, wheat germ, sausage, cheese, chicken, turkey, duck, rice, ricotta cheese, and cottage cheese.

Lysine

Lysine is an essential amino acid, and must be obtained by the diet, as it cannot be produced by the human body. Lysine is found in large amounts in the muscles. In the body lysine is a critical protein required for growth, tissue repair, and production of hormones, enzymes, antibodies, and maintenance of lean body mass. Additionally, it helps reduce the incidence of herpes outbreaks.

Lysine is effective against herpes because it reduces viral growth in both Type I and Type II herpes simplex. Type I herpes simplex involves the mouth causing cold sores or fever blisters in the area. Type II or HSV-2 involves the genital area and causes painful lesions. Type II herpes is considered a sexually transmitted disease and may be spread through any skin-to-skin contact.

Herpes zoster virus causes shingles or the painful blisters that occur usually along the rib cage. Lysine suppresses the virus by restoring the balance of nutrients retarding viral growth for all types of herpes. The proper balance of lysine to arginine ratio helps suppress the virus. (See section on herpes in Amino Acids in Therapy section, p. 167)

Lysine helps in the treatment of lead toxicity. Lysine stimulates the absorption of calcium and reduces calcium loss that helps with osteoporosis. Lysine plays a key part in the formation of collagen and stabilizes collagen. The growth and repair of muscle tissue involves lysine. Collagen is essential for the consistency of bone and connective tissues such as cartilage, tendons, and skin. Supplementing with additional L-Lysine helps adults suffering from osteoporosis by enhancing the absorption of calcium from the intestines and preventing the loss of calcium in the urea cycle. Supplemental lysine facilitates mineral bone density that prevents further bone loss in patients where this is an issue. Research indicates that lysine when combined with arginine assists in the formation of collagen and boosts the bone manufacturing cells.

Lysine is the precursor to carnitine, an amino acid that plays a role in fat regulation, cholesterol, and cardiovascular diseases. Lysine stimulates carnitine synthesis. As aging occurs an accumulation of lead and other heavy metals often happens. Lysine helps remove lead and other heavy metals. For maximum absorption of lysine, Vitamin B6 must be present.

Symptoms of lysine deficiency include fatigue, inability to concentrate, irritability, bloodshot eyes, retarded growth, anemia, hair loss, and reproductive problems.

Good food sources of lysine include yeast, parsley, soy, beef, pork, lamb, eggs, cheese, gelatins, lima beans, milk and dairy. Cereals, rice, millet, wheat, and sesame seeds contain very little lysine. Amounts required for optimum health varies widely from person to person from 500 to 1,600 mg per day, depending on their particular biochemistry. If outbreaks of herpes occur, increase the amount to 3,000 mg daily, until outbreak subsides.

Methionine

Methionine, an essential amino acid, represents one of the sulfur containing amino acids. Methionine is a methyl donor, critical for the formation of many important substances such as nucleic acids, epinephrine, choline, lecithin, carnitine, melatonin, collagen, serine, creatine, and deanol. Additionally, methionine can be a detoxifying agent assisting the removal from the body of heavy metals such as lead. Methionine stimulates the formation of glutathione that helps neutralize toxins and helps with acetaminophen or methotrexate poisoning. When methionine is given within 10 hours after acetaminophen or methotrexate poisoning, it effectively treats severe liver damage.

Methionine is necessary for selenium to be absorbed and utilized in the body. As an antioxidant, it protects the body from effects of radiation. Normal metabolism of homocysteine require B6 and methionine. Excess homocysteine can cause plaque formation in the arteries, leading to cardiovascular disease. If supplementing with methionine, always add B6 and folic acid to prevent a buildup of homocysteine. Methionine can be synthesized into cysteine, cystine, and taurine, if sulfur is present.

Excess methionine has been suggested in one type of schizophrenia, while low levels are seen with depression. Supplementing with methionine helps lower histamine levels in the body, and sufferers of allergies, asthma, and chronic pain may find methionine supplementation helpful. Heroin addicts often have low pain thresholds and high histamine levels. Methionine lowers the excess histamine levels usually present during heroin, amphetamine, or barbiturate withdrawal. In some depressed patients, methionine lifts depression with supplementation of 1 gram of methionine, morning and evening. Compared to MAO inhibitor antidepressants, methionine proves more effective. Patients with liver disease, HIV/AIDS, Parkinson's disease, or pancreatitis are higher risks for developing a methionine deficiency. Methionine (2 grams /day) along with several antioxidants reduced the pain and reoccurrences of pancreatitis in a small, but well controlled study.

Supplementing with too much methionine for a long

time produces upset stomach and vomiting. Diets high in methionine increase cholesterol and homocysteine levels that potentials the risk of heart disease and stroke. Usual supplemental dosage of methionine is 800 to 1,000 mg per day.

Food sources for methionine include seaweed (kelp), sunflowers, fish, dairy products, beans, beef, pork, chicken, wild game, eggs, lentils, onions, pumpkin and sesame seeds, soybeans, nuts, avocado, broccoli, cauliflower, mushrooms, potatoes, spinach, green peas, peanuts, pistachio, macadamia nuts, cooked corn, cottage cheese, cheese, and wheat germ.

SAMe
S-Adenosyl Methionine

Recently, reports about SAMe (S-Adenosyl Methionine) abound for the treatment of depression. SAMe became commercially available in the U.S. in 1999. SAMe derives from methionine and adenosine triphosphate (ATP). The compound of SAMe is very unstable and requires refrigeration from the manufacturing phase to the finished capsule in the bottle.

Oral absorption of SAMe is less than 1%, so it is not very bioavailable to the body. In one study, only 71% of the patients treated with oral SAMe increased their serum SAMe concentrations. Most studies done with SAMe used the parenteral (injection) form. The average adult makes between 7 to 8 grams of SAMe a day.

Patients with a history of mania, or bipolar disorder, should not use SAMe. Also, the safety of its use by heart or coronary patients remains questionable. SAMe transforms into homocysteine. It is unknown if SAMe increases the homocysteine levels in the body or influences the development of heart disease. Side effects from SAMe include nausea, mania, forced speech, and the display of grandiose ideas. Dr. Phyllis Bronson of the Aspen Clinic, reports that some patients feel extremely irritable because SAMe impacts their levels of dopamine. She advises patients to work with their individual biochemistry. Individuals with high serum methionine (per amino acid analysis), taking psychotropic (such as thorazine or haldol) or SSRI (Selective Serotonin Reuptake Inhibitors) or SNRI (Serotonin Norepinephrine Reuptake Inhibitors) medications, may experience temporary psychosis or extreme agitation after taking SAMe. Increased risk of Serotonin Syndrome is a possibility if SAMe is combined with MAOIs, SSRIs, or SNRIs. High serotonin levels cause Serotonin Syndrome with symptoms such as anxiety, restlessness, muscle tremors and twitches. The only treatment for Serotonin Syndrome is time.

The dosage of SAMe is usually 800 mg, twice daily, taken on an empty stomach. SAMe is very expensive compared to other supplements and drugs. The average cost of a month's supply of SAMe is $250. At the Pain & Stress Center, combining (Super Balanced Neurotransmitter Complex®) with methionine proves more effective than SAMe. This better-than-SAMe combination is stable and much less expensive for the treatment of depression. If you combine methionine with SBNC, you supply your brain with all the neurotransmitters it needs to make SAMe. Your body knows how much SAMe is right for you and will manufacture all the SAMe it needs. If you weigh less than 150 pounds, use two in the morning and 1500 milligrams of methionine, twice daily. If you weigh more than 150 pounds, use two capsules in the morning and afternoon, along with 1500 mg methionine, twice daily. Add 150 mg of timed-release B6, to activate the amino acids.

SAMe proves helpful with osteoarthritis patients since it stimulates the formation of proteoglycans (glucoproteins with a high polysaccharide content) that are used for cartilage regeneration. SAMe has anti-inflammatory effects and analgesic effects.

Ornithine

Ornithine is a non-essential amino acid that can be synthesized from arginine via urea cycle pathways. Ornithine is the precursor to arginine, glutamine, and citrulline and later proline and hydroxyproline. When taken by mouth, ornithine has actions similar to arginine and citrulline. Lysine inhibits the absorption of ornithine.

Ornithine is involved in metabolism of ammonia and its removal. Ornithine stimulates release of growth hormone, supports wound healing, and promotes liver regeneration. Insufficient protein intake or poor nourishment may cause low levels of ornithine. Low levels of ornithine are seen in patients with overall low amino acid levels such as institutionalized patients or patients with inborn growth or genetic defects such as PKU (phenylketonuria), patients with depression or chronic illness. With liver (hepatic) failure or higher than normal ammonia loads, higher levels of ornithine will exist.

Athletes often combine ornithine with arginine and carnitine to stimulate muscle mass while decreasing fat. These amino acids are thought to boost human growth hormone (HGH) promoting muscular growth. Body builders often supplement with 1,500 to 2,500 mg of ornithine twice daily to stimulate human growth hormone. Dosages in this range may cause insomnia. Children should not use ornithine until they have fully grown to their adult height. Excess growth hormones causes coarse and thickened skin; this is reversible when excess is removed. Too much growth hormone over a long period of time triggers irreversible enlargement of the joints, lowers the voice pitch, and may cause a pituitary form of diabetes.

Ornithine alpha-ketoglutarate (OKG) is a combination of ornithine and glutamine and is conditionally essential. During times of severe stress such as surgery or after trauma such as severe burns or injury, the body cannot manufacture enough OKG. When a catabolic state exists in the body, it breaks down body proteins to steal the needed amino acids. The body fails to use proteins from the diet and elevated levels of protein breakdown by-products show up in the urine when the body goes into a catabolic state. Studies of hospitalized patients recuperating from severe injuries or illnesses demonstrate that OKG blocks the catabolic effects of cortisone while directly stimulating an anabolic (builds up) state. OKG is given both orally or intravenously to burn, trauma, surgical, the elderly or chronically malnourished patients. Increased HGH may occur from OKG with doses of 12 mg per day intravenously, but doctors use doses of 20 to 30 grams per day on burn or trauma patients. These patients have shorter hospitalizations and fewer fatalities. High dose OKG (over 5 to 10 grams) may cause diarrhea and stomach cramps. Pregnant or nursing woman should avoid OKG. Caution should be used with high dose OKG.

Phenylalanine

Phenylalanine, an essential amino acid, functions as the parent substance, or precursor of tyrosine. Phenylalanine converts to tyrosine in the liver.

Phenylalanine Pathway

Phenylalanine ➞ Tyrosine ➞ Dopamine ➞ Norepinephrine
↓
Epinephrine

Phenylketonurics (PKU) cannot convert phenylalanine into tyrosine because PKUs lack the enzyme, phenylalanine hydroxylase.

The formation of thyroid hormone requires phenylalanine. Although phenylalanine is not found in the brain, it resides in many brain peptides, proteins, and neurotransmitters. Phenylalanine is the raw substance that produces several compounds of the catecholamine family responsible for the transmission of nerve impulses, assuming an adequate supply of phenylalanine. Norepinephrine, a major neurotransmitter, derives from tyrosine or phenylalanine. The amount of norepinephrine available to the brain is predisposed by the amount of phenylalanine or tyrosine available. Phenylalanine is one of the few amino acids readily converted into brain compounds like norepinephrine that control a person's mood. Phenylalanine or tyrosine, helps give a positive, uplifting effect on mood, alertness, and ambition. Often, this amino acid is deficient in depressed people. Phenylalanine can also stimulate the release of CCK (cholecystokinin) that, in effect, turns off the appetite.

Other phenylalanine derivatives such as epinephrine are excreted at the nerve terminals in the hypothalamus, and norepinephrine is excreted at the sympathetic nerve endings, giving rise to the fight-or-flight response. Norepinephrine is stored in presynaptic vesicles in certain central synapses. During times of stress, the body's adrenal glands are under immense pressure to produce epinephrine and norepinephrine. Often, they become low or depleted. This depletion can lead to depression and stress which can cause pain, anxiety, uncertainty, and fear.

Supplementing with phenylalanine or tyrosine helps increase the level of norepinephrine in the brain. Many antidepressants work by increasing or manipulating the norepinephrine level in the brain. Often the drugs work by blocking the norepinephrine from re-entering the vesicles or pouches found at the synapse. The natural way to normalize the brain levels of norepinephrine is with supplementation of tyrosine or phenylalanine. Therapeutic dosage ranges from 500 to 1,500 mg per day. Phenylalanine should be used with extreme caution in hypertensive patients; and always take with food. People taking MAO inhibitors or tricyclic antidepressants should not use phenylalanine or tyrosine.

The DL-form of phenylalanine, or DLPA, was found to be effective in the treatment of pain, and for the depression resulting from the pain. DLPA increases the production of PEA, norepinephrine, and endorphins. PEA is a neurotransmitter-type substance with structural resemblance to amphetamine, a stimulant drug. Endorphins are the morphine-like neurotransmitters that decrease pain and give a sense of well-being. DLPA increases endorphins by preventing the breakdown of the endorphins in the brain, so they remain there longer. If you use DLPA, the suggested amount is 750 mg, four times daily.

Food sources of phenylalanine include dairy products such as cottage cheese, milk, other cheeses; meat such as chicken, turkey, and duck; and pecans, sesame seeds, lima beans, and lentils.

Therapeutic dosages of DLPA range from 500 to 3,000 mg per day, divided.

Proline

As a non-essential amino acid, proline is required for the formation of collagen; but Vitamin C must be present. The body can manufacture proline from ornithine or glutamic acid and, if needed, the body can convert it back into ornithine.

Elevation of proline may be found in alcoholics with cirrhosis, and in some patients with depression or seizure disorders. Convulsions, elevated blood calcium levels, and osteoporosis may be caused by excess proline from a genetic error.

Good food sources of proline include cottage, ricotta and other cheeses, soy, cabbage, bamboo shoots, beef, ostrich, fish, yogurt, gelatins, milk, egg whites, wheat germ, turkey, duck, seaweed, spirulina, asparagus, soy sauce, horseradish, parsley, and kidney beans.

Supplemental dose ranges from 500 to 1,000 mg, with Vitamin C.

Serine

Serine, a non-essential amino acid, is synthesized from glycine with the presence of folic acid and B6. Serine is involved in DNA synthesis. Serine, in combination with carbohydrates, may form glycoproteins. As an immunosuppressive, serine may possibly be helpful in auto-immune diseases. Serine is required for the formation of choline, ethanolamine, phospholipids and sarcosine necessary for the formation of neurotransmitters, and to stabilize cell membranes. Phospholipids are made from phosphatidylserine, and requires the presence of methionine and folic acid. Excess serine may cause psychosis and elevation of blood pressure.

Phosphatidylserine (PS) is a component of brain cell membranes. Studies support phosphatidylserine's importance in brain functions such as memory and alertness, as well as enhanced function of the aging brain. Often, aging involves alteration of structure and biochemical changes within the brain. These include changes in neuronal membrane lipid makeup and enzyme activity, reduced production and metabolism of neurotransmitters, and loss of nerve synaptic connections. In one study, 35 patients (19 males and 16 females) with prevalent involvement of mental functions associated with behavioral changes, were treated with PS (300 mg, daily) for a period of two months. The therapeutic activity of PS was evaluated through neuropsychological tests and behavioral rating scales. Results demonstrated PS was a beneficial treatment for mild to moderate deterioration of cognitive function. Another study involved probable Alzheimer's disease patients. The study confirmed that PS treated patients improved several cognitive functions; and suggested early stage Alzheimer's patients may benefit most from PS supplementation with a dosage of 100 mg, three times, daily.

Good food sources include cottage and ricotta cheeses, wheat, wheat germ, pork, luncheon meat, turkey, sausage, peanuts, and soy.

Taurine

Taurine is now classified as a conditionally essential amino acid in the adult; but in infants and children, taurine is an essential amino acid and must be obtained from the diet for normal brain development. In the developing brain, the concentration of taurine is four times that of the adult brain. Some scientists hypothesize that taurine deficiency may cause sudden-infant-death syndrome.

Taurine is a major inhibitory, sulfur amino acid. Research demonstrates these substances are involved in the functions of the cerebral cortex, cerebellum, hippocampus, hypothalamus, and in spinal and retinal neurons. Taurine in the adult is synthesized from cysteine and methionine, provided B6 and some zinc are present. Taurine is found throughout the body abundantly in the heart muscle, olfactory bulb, central nervous system, and brain—specifically the hippocampus and pineal gland. Taurine participates in a multitude of functions in the body involving the gallbladder, brain, heart, eyes, and vascular systems. As a major inhibitory amino acid, taurine's structure closely resembles the structure and metabolism of the other inhibitory neurotransmitters, GABA and glycine.

In the heart, taurine is the most concentrated amino acid. Taurine modulates heart muscular contractility and rhythms. Taurine plays a part in calcium metabolism in the heart. Taurine affects the admission of calcium into the heart-muscle cells where it is necessary for nerve impulses (heart rhythms), and helps with arrhythmias of all kinds. Some studies suggest taurine may increase the survival rate after a heart attack and reduce the elevation of calcium content in both aorta and heart muscles. The regulation of calcium may prevent the progression of arteriosclerosis.

When the body experiences chronic stress, the concentration of taurine increases in the heart. After a heart attack, the levels of taurine often decrease dramatically. In some cases, the levels drop to one-third the normal. The loss of intracellular taurine may contribute to arrhythmias (abnormal heartbeats) where acute ischemia (low oxygen levels within the heart muscle) occurs. In Japan, doctors are using taurine widely for all types of heart disease. When congestive heart failure occurs, the concentration of taurine increases as the body tries to naturally correct the problem metabolically. In one study, congestive heart failure (CHF) patients were given 4 grams of taurine, per day, for a month. Nineteen of the 24 patients improved. Another double blind crossover study involved fourteen patients. The patients were given 6 grams of taurine, or a placebo, in additional to conventional treatment in a randomized crossover design for four weeks, with a two-week washout period in-between. Eleven of the fourteen or 78% improved on taurine compared to twenty-one percent, or three of fourteen, on the placebo. While on the placebo, the heart-failure scores did not change appreciably, but the heart-failure scores decreased significantly for the patients on taurine. Additionally, during the taurine administration, no patient worsened, whereas four placebo patients did get worse. Taurine seems to assist in CHF by acting as a diuretic, ridding the body of excess water and sodium, and as a heart stimulator with doses of 2 grams per day. Taurine and magnesium levels drop dramatically whenever heart arrhythmias occur, and replenishing both assists in controlling heart arrhythmias. Taurine helps prevent the decrease of potassium within the cells of the heart. Decreased potassium causes electrical instability, leading to heart arrhythmias. Additionally, taurine helps balance the calcium and potassium levels in the heart.

Normal brain development in infants requires taurine. It protects and stabilizes the brain's fragile cell membranes. Taurine acts as an inhibitory neurotransmitter in the brain, like the neurotransmitters, GABA and glycine. In the brain, the site of greatest seizure activity, researchers found low taurine concentrations. Taurine proves effective in the treatment of epilepsy, acting as an anticonvulsant. The levels are lower than normal for over half of the amino acids, if epilepsy is present; but the levels of taurine are higher than normal, except in the cerebrospinal fluid. The usual dosage of taurine for epilepsy is 3,000 mg per day with a non-protein meal. Taurine helps people with tics or other spastic conditions. As a word of caution, taurine should not be taken simultaneously with aspirin or any salicylates because taurine may increase the release of stomach acid.

In patients with tics, twitches, or spastic conditions, taurine proves helpful. In her book, *Tired or Toxic,* Dr. Sherry Rogers reports the tics of Tourette's syndrome as abnormal firings of the nervous system. Research on Tourette's points to multiple triggers, but taurine assists in reducing the tics. The usual dosage for tics is 1,000 mg, twice to three times per day. With Tourette's syndrome, supplementation with other amino acids and nutrients is extremely important. Research shows taurine helps reduce muscular spasms/rigidity in patients with muscular dystrophy.

A deficiency of taurine exists in patients with depression. If a depressed patient is environmentally sensitive, a taurine deficiency can compound chemical sensitivities, and decrease the body's ability to detoxify chemicals.

Taurine is present in the eye in high concentrations, and most abundant of the amino acids in the eye. In retinitis pigmentosa, Dr. Voaden found abnormally low blood levels of taurine.

Taurine is necessary for the formation of one of the bile acids and for proper functioning of the gallbladder. Taurine, in doses of three to six grams daily, divided, increases bile production, which may prevent the formation of gallstones. The bile may be a route of excretion of chemicals detoxified by the body. Taurine is sometimes called upon to help control inflammation or infection.

Taurine, or a modified taurine, may someday supersede synthetic tranquilizers. Stress depletes the body of taurine. Whenever you experience more than usual amounts of stress, chronically, or if you have an illness, the need for taurine increases. Chronic pain of any kind depletes the body of taurine. Often, supplementation is necessary, as the need for taurine is greater than what we can obtain from our diets. In over 300 amino acid profiles done on patients at the Pain & Stress Center, nine out of ten patients showed a deficiency of taurine. In most cases, one to three grams of taurine supplementation was required daily.

Best food sources of taurine include meats, especially organ meats, and fish. Supplementation is necessary, as the taurine need becomes greater than what can be obtained from the diet, alone.

Usual dosage of taurine is 500 to 3,000 mg per day,

preferably on an empty stomach. Women require more taurine than men, since men have higher enzyme levels.

Our pets (domestic dogs and cats) need taurine, too. Most pets are dependent upon their diet for taurine, but taurine is often absent in commercially prepared foods. A deficiency of taurine causes degeneration of the retina of the eye, often leading to blindness. To ensure your pet obtains enough taurine, supplement the diet part of the time with fresh meat (organ meats, liver, kidney, brains, heart) or fish and supplementing with taurine powder or capsules. These foods are the best sources of taurine for pets.

Theanine

Recently, L-Theanine has come to the forefront. In 1949 Japanese chemists discovered l-theanine from green tea leaves. Green tea has been used for thousands of years and research studies documents theanine's safety. Theanine appears to play a role in the creation of the major inhibitory neurotransmitter, GABA. But Theanine influences not only GABA, but dopamine and serotonin. A study published in the *Journal of Food Science and Technology* confirms theanine has a significant effect on the neurotransmitter release of dopamine and serotonin. Dopamine is the feel good chemical in the brain while serotonin calms, uplifts mood, and decreases pain.

Clinical research documents that theanine creates a sense of well-being, calm, and relaxation, but has many other benefits as well. Theanine stimulates the production of alpha waves in the brain. The human brain continuously produces weak electrical pulses that form brain waves. Four different types of brain waves are classified according to frequency; they are alpha, beta, delta, and theta brain waves. Alpha waves indicate relaxed wakefulness in the brain. Beta waves show a state of wakeful anxiety, rapid pulse, and expected stress. Theta brain waves indicate a relaxed state followed by dozing sleep. Delta waves are slow brain waves that indicate deep sleep. Each brain wave relates to your state of mind and overall mental state. Every time your mood changes, your brain waves change along with your blood pressure, heart rate, and body rhythms.

Deep meditation produces a state of deep relaxation with alpha waves present in the brain. If alpha waves are present, the brain is less vulnerable to the effects of stress. Scientists have been searching for ways to create an alpha state of mind without using psychoactive drugs. Theanine is an answer! Theanine initiates a mellow mood, evens temper, while enhancing focus and concentration. Thirty to forty minutes after ingesting theanine in capsule form, your mood mellows indicating the alpha state is beginning. Your muscles follow suit as your brain changes gears. Theanine stimulates the production of alpha waves signaling your brain to relax, but you are mentally alert without drowsiness. Theanine does not produce theta waves so you do not experience any negative side effects while driving or working. You remain alert and in control. You think more clearly without any dull feelings and are actually more productive. Theanine can be taken anytime and food consumption does not affect it. Theanine does counter the effects of caffeine.

Theanine converts to GABA in the brain making theanine an excellent choice for anyone with anxiety/stress and phobias. When the brain is in an alpha state, anxiety and fear message from the amygdala cannot overwhelm the cortex (brain). The amygdala stores all fear stimuli and is the emotional storehouse of anxiety related messages in the brain. The amygdala releases these stored stimuli during stressful times. In 1999 researchers at the University of Shizuoka in Shizuoka, Japan confirmed theanine's unique properties. Their research found that theanine facilitates relaxation, but helps control hypertension (high blood pressure), enhances learning while increasing mental acuity and concentration as well as supporting the immune system.

A food source of theanine is green tea. The usual dosage of L-Theanine (L–T®) is 200 mg, three to four times per day, divided for adults; children over 6 years of age can use theanine, but start with 100 mg, twice daily. The capsule form of theanine gives the benefits of theanine without the caffeine. You must drink 4 to 5 cups of green tea to equal 500 mg of green tea extract. A decaffeinated green tea extract with 95% EGCG (polyphenols) in capsule form provides the benefits of green tea and is readily available.

For complete information about theanine and green tea, read my books entitled *Theanine, The Relaxation Amino Acid* and *Green Tea, Healing Miracle*.

Threonine

Threonine is an essential amino acid, and is the precursor to brain glycine. The body requires threonine for proper digestion, intestinal tract function, and for formation of collagen, elastin, and tooth enamel. Threonine breaks down into glucose, and into the amino acids glycine and serine. The highest concentration of threonine are found in the heart, central nervous system, and skeletal muscles.

Threonine stimulates the thymus gland and stimulates the immune system including the production of antibodies. It is important for liver health and plays a lesser role in preventing fat accumulation in the liver. Vegans are at highest risk for a threonine deficiency due to the low levels of threonine in vegetables and grains. A deficiency of threonine suppresses the immune system.

Threonine has proven helpful in multiple sclerosis, Lou Gehrig's disease (ALS), other nervous system conditions and in some patients with agitated depression and mania. Threonine levels decline with age, and increase during stressful times or severe trauma such as accident or burn patients. In these patients threonine urinary excretion levels increase and may require supplementation to assist recovery. Though threonine toxicities are rare, long term excessive intake may cause hypertension.

Good food sources includes seaweed (kelp), sesame and sunflower seeds, soy, eggs, milk, beef, beans, nuts, pork, turkey, wheat germ, cottage and ricotta cheeses.

Tryptophan

Tryptophan is an essential amino acid, and must be obtained in the diet. It ultimately breaks down into serotonin, the calming neurotransmitter in the brain. Serotonin helps us feel calm, relaxed, and in control.

Tryptophan Pathway
Tryptophan → 5-HTP → Serotonin

Tryptophan is a precursor of serotonin, melatonin, and niacin. Serotonin is synthesized from tryptophan. Serotonin is a brain neurotransmitter, platelet-clotting factor, and neurohormone found in the organs throughout the body. Tryptophan is essential in maintaining the body's protein balance. When food that is protein deficient or lacking tryptophan is fed to growing or mature individuals, such foods fail to replace worn-out materials lost by the body during the organic activities of its cells, tissues, and organs. The amino acid, tryptophan, is exhausted by the vital activities of the body and, in turn, must be replaced to prevent atrophy of the body's structures.

One of the few substances capable of passing the blood-brain barrier, tryptophan plays a variety of important roles in mental activity. When tryptophan intake is deficient, especially during periods of stress, serotonin levels drop causing depression, anxiety, insecurity, hyperactivity, insomnia, and pain. The body requires ample supplies of Vitamin B6 for the formation of tryptophan.

Tryptophan's role in behavior has been demonstrated by the number of mental functions it directly influences. Serotonin produces a relaxed, calm, secure, mellow, and morphine-like analgesic feeling. Only 1 to 2% of all serotonin in the body is found in the brain. Hyperactive children/adults have a low serotonin level. Aggression reflects one of the most widely recognized signs of reduced serotonin. Supplements containing tryptophan and Vitamin B6 can correct some of the biochemical disorders related to aggression.

Another significant finding in studies done with tryptophan demonstrated that low levels of serotonin could play a part in the development of depression. Combining tryptophan (1,000 mg) with tyrosine in doses of 3,000 mg per day, at bedtime, can mimic the effects of most antidepressants. Tryptophan is useful in unipolar depression or constant, low-grade depression with no highs or lows.

Both depression and pain can have profound effects on a person's ability to fall asleep. Difficulty in falling asleep can be caused by low serotonin levels. But tryptophan has been shown to effectively solve insomnia problems, reducing the time needed to fall asleep, and increasing the number of hours spent sleeping. The usual dosage is 500 to 1,000 mg, taken one hour prior to bedtime with a carbohydrate such as orange juice or fruit.

Because serotonin is a neurotransmitter and neurohormone, it is one of the most important chemicals to help control moods. Best of all, tryptophan is safe, and is a natural relaxant and tranquilizer of the central nervous system. The body has no difficulty in rapidly metabolizing and clearing it from the body. As an essential amino acid necessary for life, tryptophan is the sole precursor for serotonin. It does not simply pass through the gut into the brain, to become serotonin. It must compete with five other amino acids—tyrosine, phenylalanine, leucine, isoleucine, and valine—at the blood-brain barrier. In order to increase the amount of brain serotonin, the ratio of tryptophan must be elevated out of proportion to the competing amino acids. Metabolism and protein intake may alter this ratio.

About 90% of serum tryptophan is bound to albumin. Free fatty acids (serum) share the same albumin binding sites. Changing both the blood sugar level and insulin may increase and decrease the proportion of free tryptophan that has access to the brain. In the total serum amino acid profile, the ratio of tryptophan to the nutrient amino acids has been elevated in each instance. Tyrosine has also been elevated in each instance. About 1% of ingested tryptophan metabolizes to serotonin. About 90% of the tryptophan metabolizes through kynurenic acid to nicotinic acid.

The neurotransmitters directly depend on dietary tryptophan and other amino acids. Circadian rhythms effect the amino acid utilization in the nervous system. Circadian rhythm is a specific type of periodicity for the uptake and utilization of substances. This has recently been shown with use of tryptophan in the treatment of insomnia. When tryptophan is used during the day, it does not seem to induce sleep, only a calm, relaxed state; but when taken near bedtime, it seems to induce sleep, as shown in sleep studies done at several medical centers. This seems to indicate that tryptophan's uptake across the blood-brain barrier corresponds to the circadian rhythms of the sleep cycle. Its absorption and conversion in the brain to serotonin more effectively occurs during times when a person would normally sleep. This is why it is clinically suggested to administer tryptophan at bedtime, if used for treating sleep disorders. Conversely, tryptophan or tyrosine should be used during the day to treat certain forms of depression. Liquid homeopathic serotonin used 3 to 4 times daily will elevate the serotonin level. Melatonin also elevates the serotonin level, and is effective for sleep problems. Melatonin is produced by the pineal gland in the brain, and is a neurohormone.

Two researchers in England compared the antidepressant effects of tryptophan and Tofranil. Tofranil, or imipramine, is a drug commonly used for depression. Both groups of patients with depression improved. The study revealed that tryptophan was just as effective as the laboratory-produced drug, and there were no side effects from the tryptophan. Conversely, the side effects for the Tofranil group included blurring of vision, dryness of the mouth, low blood pressure, urinary retention, heart palpitations, hepatitis, and seizures.

Tryptophan is obtained in the diet every day. Many rich natural forms of tryptophan include: bananas, green leafy vegetables, red meat, pork, turkey, dairy products, pineapple, avocados, eggs, soy, sesame and pumpkin seeds, and lentils. Large doses of tryptophan, when combined with niacinamide and Vitamin B6, can enhance the conversion of tryptophan to serotonin.

Currently, tryptophan is available selectively, but the authors feel 5-HTP is more effective because it is one step closer to converting to serotonin. But the cost of tryptophan is high. Tryptophan was removed for sale in 1989 because of a contaminated-batch that caused EMS (eosinophilia-myalgia syndrome). The F.D.A. determined the cause was tryptophan and not the contaminated batch. F.D.A. reclassified tryptophan as an unapproved experimental drug, and ordered recall of all products except where tryptophan occurred naturally.

But within the last several years, 5-HTP, or 5-hydroxytryptophan, has become available. 5-HTP derives from griffonia seeds, a member of the legume or bean family. 5-HTP, about 10 times stronger than tryptophan, readily converts to serotonin. Suggested dosage is 50 to 300 mg of 5-HTP, daily.

One study compared 5-HTP to Luvox, an antidepressant. Subjects with depression were given 100 mg of 5-HTP, three times daily, or 150 mg, of Luvox, three times daily. Evaluations were done at 2, 4, and 6 weeks. After 2 weeks, both groups reported a significant reduction in depression. By week 4, 15 of 36 5-HTP patients and 18 of 33 Luvox patients reported at least a 50% improvement in depression symptoms. Final assessment demonstrated the 5-HTP patients had the greatest improvement and the least amount of treatment failures. Another study involving endogenous depression (arising from within the individual, in all likelihood genetic) demonstrated marked improvement or cure in 69% of patients receiving 5-HTP.

Note: *Tryptophan or 5-HTP should not be taken with SSRIs (Selective Serotonin Reuptake Inhibitors) or SNRI (Serotonin Norepinephrine Reuptake Inhibitor) drugs such as Prozac, Paxil, Luvox, or Effexor.*

Tyrosine

Tyrosine is the first breakdown product of phenylalanine, and is considered a non-essential amino acid because the body can make it from phenylalanine. Tyrosine is the stress amino acid.

Dr. Gelenberg, at Harvard Medical School, determined tyrosine is more effective than antidepressants for relief of depression. To rapidly increase the norepinephrine level, use tyrosine. Because it is one step closer to norepinephrine, you feel the effect more rapidly. Suggested amount of tyrosine is one 850 mg capsule of pharmaceutical grade tyrosine, three times daily. *Do not take tyrosine with MAO inhibitors or tricyclic antidepressants, if you have schizophrenia or a history of melanoma.*

Researchers at Urije University, in the Netherlands, found supplementing with tyrosine enhanced memory and reduced blood pressure in healthy, young, military cadets. The cadets received either protein-rich drinks containing two grams tyrosine, or carbohydrate-rich drinks with equal calories. After six days, the supplemented cadets performed better on memory and tracking tests, and showed decreased systolic blood pressures. Researchers concluded that tyrosine supplementation might, under working conditions distinguished by psychosocial and physical stress, reduce the effects of stress and fatigue.

See the phenylalanine section for metabolism and specifics.

S.B.N.C.
Super Balanced Neurotransmitter Complex

The brain communicates through neurotransmitters, the chemical language of the brain. A super balanced neurotransmitter complex contains the amino acids in a special blend that nourishes the brain. An unbalanced diet, anxiety, chronic pain, depression, and grief, plus other factors, contribute to disturbances in amino acid metabolism. S.B.N.C. contains the special amino acid mix of glutamine, GABA, taurine, phenylalanine, glycine, arginine, methionine, valine, lysine, leucine, alanine, isoleucine, histidine, and pyridoxal 5'phosphate (B6). These 14 amino acids, plus the activating agent, B6, can be taken on a daily basis without fear of creating an amino acid imbalance. S.B.N.C. can be combined with other amino

Disorders Associated with Amino Acid Imbalances

- ADD/ADHD
- Alcoholism
- Ammonia toxicity
- Ataxia (defective muscular coordination)
- Behavioral disorders
- Cardiovascular disease
- Chemical intolerances
- Chronic fatigue
- Chronic gastrointestinal distress or bowel irregularity
- Depression
- Dermatitis (inflammation of the skin)
- Detoxification impairments
- Excessive inflammation
- Failure to thrive (infancy)
- Family history or early symptoms of degenerative disease
- Frequent headaches
- Frequent infections and persistent inflammatory responses
- Hyperlipidemia (high blood lipid levels)
- Hypertension (high blood pressure)
- Hypotonia (loss of muscle tone)
- Inflammatory disorders
- Impaired mental development
- Insomnia
- Intolerances (persistent) to foods and chemicals
- Mental confusion
- Mental retardation
- Myopathies (muscular diseases)
- Neurological disorders
- Neural tube defects (birth defects)
- Ocular disorders (eye)
- Osteoporosis
- Oxidative stress
- Poor immunity
- Poor wound healing
- Rheumatoid arthritis
- Seizures
- Short stature or chronically underweight, growth failure (children)
- Weak skin and nails

Source: *Diagnostic Value of Amino Acid Analysis*, Great Smokies Diagnostic Laboratory.

acids for a total orthomolecular approach.

Research has shown substantial improvement in chronic fatigue patients using the S.B.N.C. Complex, CoEnzyme Q10, Alpha KG, and Mag Link. S.B.N.C. should be taken on a daily basis to correct impairments in biochemistry that can either cause or complicate health conditions. Amino acids, because of their intimate involvement in metabolic regulation, prove very useful therapeutic agents that reverse biochemical impairments related to amino acid metabolism. S.B.N.C. has been instrumental in correcting mental and stress-related disturbances, food and chemical intolerances, learning disabilities, frequent headaches, fibromyalgia, chronic fatigue, mental and emotional disturbances, hyperactivity, and some neurological disorders. S.B.N.C. is available in capsule form. When withdrawing from various drugs, use S.B.N.C. to increase neurotransmitters in the brain and body. Dosage is usually two S.B.N.C., twice daily to restore brain chemistry; for those over 200 pounds, use three S.B.N.C. twice daily. S.B.N.C. can be used safely while withdrawing from medications.

Amino Acid Cofactors

B6 Pyridoxine

Due to its function in the body, B6 is one of the most important vitamins the body needs. B6 transforms to pyridoxal 5'phosphate, or P5'P. P5'P is a coenzyme that activates enzymes and enzyme systems. Our bodies could not function without enzymes because they trigger every chemical reaction within the body. One hundred eighteen enzymes and nineteen of the twenty amino acids rely on Vitamin B6. B6 serves as a catalyst for the enzymes in the body, and without it we could not digest amino acids (proteins), carbohydrates, and fats. B6 is necessary for life. B6 and magnesium are necessary cofactors for proper brain function.

At Tufts University a study by the U.S. Department of Agriculture Human Nutrition Research Center on Aging, revealed the elderly need at least 3 milligrams of Vitamin B6, daily. B6 should not be taken in dosages greater than 300 mg, per day. Daily ingestion of over 300 mg of B6 can cause irreversible neurotoxicity. Neurotoxicity involves dosages of B6 too high or toxic to the nerves in the dorsal root ganglia (spinal cord) and to sensory nerves in the

---

U.S. Recommended Daily Value Allowance (USDV) for B6

0.3 milligrams, for infants six to eleven months old;

1 milligram, for children nine to thirteen years of age;

1.5 milligrams, for females fourteen to eighteen years of age;

1.7 milligrams, for males fourteen to eighteen years of age;

2.2 milligrams, for pregnant women;

2 milligrams, for adult males.

Signs and Symptoms of Vitamin B6 Deficiency in the Human Body

- Paresthesia (pins-and-needles numbness and tingling in distal parts of the hands or feet)
- Impaired sensation in the fingers
- Impaired flexion of the finger joints
- Fluctuating edema in the hands
- Morning stiffness in the fingers
- Pain in the hands
- Impaired coordination of the fingers
- Weakness of pinch (the pressure point between the thumb and index finger)
- Increased tendency to drop objects
- Tenderness over the carpal tunnel with Tinel's sign (a tingling sensation radiating out into the hand and accompanied by pain at the wrist) and Phalen's sign (paresthesia in the fingers) that becomes worse when the median nerve is squeezed between the ligament and tendons while the wrist is held flexed for thirty to sixty seconds.
- Pain in the elbows or shoulders
- Pain upon movement of the thumb knuckle (metacarpophalangeal joint)
- Sleep paralysis (the temporary inability to lift the arm or hand upon awakening during the night)
- Edema from steroid-hormone therapy (a puffy swelling in the tissues of the face, hands, feet, or legs when steroid hormones, particularly when taking large doses of cortisone or female hormones such as estrogen)
- Macular edema (an abnormal collection of fluid and fatty substances that have leaked from tiny arteries near the central portion of the retina of the eye, resulting in disturbed central vision)

If you notice any of these signs and symptoms, contact your physician. You may find Vitamin B6 therapy extremely helpful.

Source: *Vitamin B6 Therapy*, by John M. Ellis, M.D. and Jean Pamplin; p. 43.

feet and legs. Dr. Karl Folkers, of Clayton Foundation, University of Texas, determined daily dosages of 50 to 300 milligrams of B6 to be safe for adults over seventeen years, including pregnant women, and patients with diabetes, heart disease, or carpal tunnel syndrome. B6 may improve or prevent acne, alcoholism, asthma, heart disease, diabetes, hyperactivity, PMS, repetitive stress injury, and pregnancy/toxemia.

The body requires B6 and four minerals, especially if you have diabetes or any diabetic complications. The four minerals comprise chromium, magnesium, zinc, and potassium. Studies demonstrate that B6 slows the development of diabetic complications such as diabetic retinopathy, kidney problems, or heart disease. Evidence suggests that diabetics who have taken 100 to 300 mg, daily, for several years, are more likely to survive a heart attack and live longer than diabetics not supplementing with B6.

B6 functions in the liver, brain, blood, muscles, cartilage, bone, hormones, arteries, etc., are still under investigation by scientists. Elevated homocysteine levels in the blood contribute to changes in arteries and the development of heart disease. At New York University Medical Center, studies proved that high levels of homocysteine and low levels of B6 contribute to severe calcification in the aortas of patients with advanced atherosclerosis. Calcified deposits promote blockage of arteries. B6 is readily destroyed with baking or other cooking. Heat destroys B6. You should take B6 as a time-released form (150 mg) that releases over eight to nine hours, or take pyridoxal-5-phosphate (P5'P), the biological form of B6.

Best food sources of B6 include whole grain cereal, potatoes, bananas, chickpeas (garbanzo beans), chicken, oatmeal, pork, beef, sunflower seeds, tomatoes, and avocados.

Timed Release Rodex Forte B6

Supplementation with timed-release B6 disperses B6 over a period of 8 to 9 hours. This timed-release B6 helps prevent neurotoxicity which can occur in doses greater than 500 mg over a prolonged period of time.

P5'P (Pyridoxal 5' Phosphate) Active B6

Pyridoxal 5' Phosphate, or P5'P, the biological (active) form of B6 is necessary for the utilization of all amino acids, proteins, fats, and carbohydrates. If P5'P is not present, increased excretion of most amino acids occurs as well as increased formation of abnormal amino acid metabolites.

Unlike B6 there is no fear of toxicity with P5'P, even in children. Reaction to MSG may indicates a deficiency of P5'P or Vitamin B6. Reactions to MSG may effectively be prevented with supplementation of B6 or P5'P.

Magnesium

Magnesium is an essential cofactor in over 300 enzyme reactions in the body. Many Americans (70%) are deficient in magnesium, and do not get enough from their diets. Magnesium and B6, or P5'P, must be present or the body cannot assimilate and properly use amino acids.

Magnesium is known as the stress mineral. As an essential cofactor in over 300 enzyme reactions that occur in the body, magnesium is necessary for energy production and DNA replication, the basis of all life. Currently, doctors emphasize calcium supplements for the prevention and treatment of osteoporosis. While trying

Magnesium/Amino Acid Connection

Symptoms of Magnesium *Deficiency*

- Anxiety
- Panic attacks
- Mitral valve prolapse
- Hypertension
- Chronic pain
- Back and neck pain
- Muscle spasms
- Migraines
- Fibromyalgia
- Spastic symptoms
- Chronic bronchitis, emphysema
- Vertigo (dizziness)
- Confusion
- Depression
- Psychosis
- Noise sensitivity
- Ringing in the ears
- Irritable-bowel syndrome
- Cardiovascular disease
- Cardiac arrhythmias
- Atherosclerosis/Intermittent claudication
- Raynaud's disease (cold hands and feet)
- TIA's (Transient Ischemic Attacks or strokes)
- Constipation
- Fatigue
- Diabetes
- Hypoglycemia
- Asthma
- Seizures
- Kidney stones
- Premenstrual syndrome
- Menstrual cramps

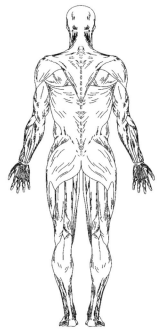

You have 657 muscles that need magnesium every second of every day. Magnesium is a cofactor for all amino acids.

For maximum benefit, add some magnesium in the form of magnesium chloride such as Mag Link or Mag Chlor 90 liquid. Try two tablets or 15 to 25 drops of Mag Chlor 90 liquid, twice to three times daily. If loose stools or diarrhea occur, decrease by one tablet or try increasing amount of time between doses. You should begin to feel a decrease in symptoms.

WARNING: People with renal or kidney failure should not take magnesium without medical supervision.

For detailed information on magnesium-deficiency symptoms, read my book, *The Anxiety Epidemic*.

to get sufficient quantities of calcium, the majority of people pay little attention to their intake of magnesium. But magnesium plays an important role in bone health.

Magnesium, like calcium, helps promote healthy bones and teeth, decreases high blood pressure, and maintains muscle health. Like calcium, magnesium is distributed throughout the body. Most magnesium is found in the bones, which store this essential mineral. A profound difference exists between calcium and magnesium at the cellular levels. Calcium concentrates outside the cell, while magnesium finds its way inside all body cells. The body needs both minerals to maintain electrical potential across the cell membranes, or simply, they assist the transmission of nerve impulses. Just as calcium is required for muscle contraction, magnesium is essential for muscle relaxation. Recent research demonstrates that humans require magnesium in a balance of 2 parts magnesium to 1 part calcium.

Until the age of 35, bone mass can increase. Bone loss occurs due to an imbalance of the mottling process, and bones begin to lose both their mineral and their gelatinous matrix. Menopause, or the change of life for a woman, usually precipitates a bone crisis. During the change-of-life years, rapid declines in bone mass occur making women more susceptible to bone fractures. Fewer fractures occur in women supplementing with magnesium and calcium than in women supplementing with only calcium. If you increase your calcium intake, it is vitally important that you also increase your intake of magnesium.

More than 50% of doctor visits are for fatigue. Modern medicine offers little for this problem. If you provide your body all the nutrients it needs for energy production, your fatigue often decreases. Magnesium proves essential for energy production in the cells. Magnesium helps relieve Chronic Fatigue Syndrome (CFS). Studies show that red-blood-cell magnesium levels measure considerably lower in CFS patients than in normal patients.

Drugs That Deplete Magnesium

Acid Blockers
•Antacids
Antibiotics
Antiviral agents
Aromatase inhibitors for Breast Cancer
Bisposphonate (bone-building drugs)
Blood pressure drugs
Cardiac glycoside (digoxin)
Central Nervous System stimulants (Ritalin)
Cholesterol agents
Corticosteroids
Hormone Replacement Therapy
Oral contraceptives
Immunosuppressants
SERMs (Selective Estrogen Receptor Modulators for breast cancer)
Sulfonamides (sulfa antibiotics, some diabetes meds)
Alcohol
Calcium supplementation (prolonged or in excess)
• Coffee
Estrogen dominance
High cortisol levels
• High sugar diet
•Malabsorption disorders (Crohn's or Celiac disease, pancreatitis, anorexia, or crash dieting)
Mineral oil

Source: *Drug Muggers* (Suzy Cohen) pp. 174-176

Magnesium deficiency causes the release of more histamine. Histamine releases whenever you react to an allergen that triggers an allergic reaction to a food, chemical, or environmental factor. Low levels of magnesium contribute to kidney stone formation. Daily supplementation with magnesium and B6 promotes removal and prevents reformation of kidney stones. A four-year study of fifty-five patients demonstrated that ingesting 500 mg of magnesium, daily, reduced by 90% the reformation of kidney stones. The control group that did not supplement with magnesium experienced a reoccurrence rate of 41%. Magnesium deficiency leads to neuromuscular malfunctions such as tremors, convulsions, high excitability, behavior disorders, neuromuscular pain, and depression. Magnesium acts as a muscle relaxant, reducing the spasms in PMS, menstrual cramps, fibromyalgia, trigger points, muscle cramps, or any other painful condition. Supplementing with magnesium chloride produces the best results.

Supplementing with magnesium is safe. Excessive magnesium occurs only in people with kidney problems or impaired kidney function. Magnesium can cause loose stools, or diarrhea, in some people. If this occurs, divide the dosage of magnesium into three to six times a day and night, or decrease by one tablet or use less drops. The best-tolerated form of magnesium is a magnesium chloride capsules, such as Mag Link or Mag Chlor 90 liquid.

The majority of healthcare practitioners do not realize that increasing intake of refined carbohydrates and processed foods increases the body's requirement for magnesium. If magnesium intake has not kept pace, subliminal deficiency occurs. Most Americans do not get enough magnesium and other vital nutrients. The percent daily value (%DV) for magnesium is 400 mg. The typical American diet provides between 200–300 mg, daily. The late Dr. Mildred Seelig, a nationally recognized magnesium specialist, estimated deficiencies in over 80 percent of the population. Reevaluate your diet and current health status, and add the needed magnesium to your supplement program. Ingestion of alcohol, soft drinks, and processed foods—all high in phosphates—cause loss of magnesium via the kidneys. Certain medications such as diuretics, asthma medications such as theophylline, being over 40 years of age, and diabetes increase the loss of magnesium from the body. Rich food sources of magnesium include whole-wheat flour, nuts—almonds, brazils, cashews, peanuts, peanut butter—green leafy vegetables, soybeans, lentils, boiled shrimp, snails, yeast, brown rice, and dried peas.

Alpha KG

Alpha KG and citric acid are elements of the Krebs cycle (TCA cycle), the chemical engine that generates energy for every cell of the body. Alpha KG works with B6 and magnesium to metabolize amino acids, thus enabling the body to convert amino acids into other substances it needs. Proper brain neurotransmitter production requires optimal amino acid metabolism. Alpha KG+ is a combination formula intended to address metabolic deficiencies seen in human plasma amino acid analyses. Alpha KG contains Alpha-Ketoglutaric acid, potassium and magnesium citrates and aspartates, B6, and Vitamin C (Ascorbyl Palmitate).

The components of Alpha KG+ work at various sites of metabolic deficiencies. When given orally, Alpha KG+ drives the Krebs cycle forward greatly enhancing cellular energy, thus decreasing fatigue and increasing stamina. Magnesium and potassium aspartates indirectly contribute to increased energy. In double-blind clinical trials, magnesium and potassium aspartates proved effective for the treatment of chronic fatigue.

Amino Acids and Metabolic Pathways

Detoxifying amino acids include cysteine, glutamine, glycine, methionine, taurine, and tyrosine.

Immuno-stimulating amino acids include alanine, aspartic acid, cysteine, glycine, lysine, and threonine.

Important Note

This section of the book divides into generalized categories by condition. Each condition includes suggested nutritional support with the most important amino acids, or combinations of amino acids (specific formulas that work), for that particular condition. To comprehensively cover certain conditions, other vitamins, herbs, or nutrients are included in this section.

Note: *You do not need to take all of the amino acids or nutrients listed.*

Pick the amino acids that apply to your symptoms, or start with a few items, and see how you feel. You can always add another amino acid or nutrient, later. If you slowly add nutrients, you will know what is helping and what is not.

Example 1. If you use the Brain Link Complex formulation that contains glutamine, you do not necessarily need to add more glutamine to your diet.

Example 2. If you have a problem with memory, start with SBNC and glutamine; then if needed, add phosphatidylserine or huperzine.

If you have questions regarding the specific supplements listed, call 1-800-669-2256 or
Visit the Pain & Stress Center web site
http://www.painstresscenter.com

Amino Acids in Therapy

Acne

Acne is a disorder of the skin that affects 80% of people aged 10 to 24 regardless of race or ethnicity. Men tend to have more severe acne than women. But acne is not limited to just teenagers. Adults into their 40s get acne. Acne results from the action of hormones on the sebaceous glands (skin's oil glands) leading to plugged pores (blackheads, whiteheads, pimples (zits) and lesions (cysts). Acne occurs on the face, neck, chest, shoulders, back, and upper arms. The sebaceous glands produce oil to lubricate the skin. If the oil becomes trapped, bacteria multiply and trigger an inflammatory response. Acne can cause severe and permanent scarring.

The exact cause of acne is unknown, but hormones, oral contraceptives, allergies, stress, consumption of processed foods, especially fried foods and sugar may contribute. Certain androgens and lithium are known to cause acne.

Remember your skin is a picture of your emotional state. For example, if you become upset or angry, within 24 to 72 hours after the incident, you experience a flare-up of acne or you have new zits appear. There is a direct relationship between your stress and your skin. Your skin reflects your emotions. If you experience a lot of stress, add the stress/anxiety amino acids (Anxiety Control, Mood Sync, Teen Link, or L–T) to help keep your brain in balance.

Suggested Nutritional Support
T–L Vite – 1 capsule with main meal.
Zinc Picolinate – 15 mg capsule with breakfast.

MSM – 500 to 1000 mg orally, twice daily.

Lysine – 500 to 1,000 mg, twice to three times daily.

Esterified Vitamin C – 1,000 mg, three times per day.

Vitamin E – 800 to 1,200 I.U. per day for 4 to 6 months, then decrease to 400 to 800 I.U. per day for maintenance.

ProDHA – 2 softgels, twice daily OR **Pure Fish Oil** – 1 softgel, twice daily. **Caution:** *Do not use if you take anticoagulants (blood thinners), are allergic to iodine, or if you will have surgery within a week.*

Decaf Green Tea Extract – 2 capsule daily.

Anxiety Control – 2 capsules twice daily, OR

Teen Link (adults, use **Mood Sync**) 2 capsules twice daily, OR use

L–T – 2 capsules twice daily. **Caution:** *If you are taking an SSRI, SNRI, tricyclic, or MAOI antidepressant, or if you have a history of a melanoma, do not use Mood Sync or Teen Link.*

First Aid Gel (Sovereign Silver) – apply topically to affected areas, if inflamed or infected, being careful not to get the silver in your eyes.

Other Factors

Keep skin and hair clean.

Avoid touching the area and don't squeeze the pimples as it inflames the skin making it more likely to become infected.

Choose cosmetics carefully, and use as little as possible.

Eat healthy foods with emphasis on fruits and vegetables. **Avoid fried or greasy foods, sugar, sodas, and caffeine.**

Addiction (Alcohol)

Alcoholism is a disease of chemical dependency. It is addictive, abusive, and eventually becomes destructive.

Alcoholism ranks with stress, mental illness, and heart disease as one of the major problems in the U.S. Alcoholism develops from a combination of factors—psychological, physiological, genetic, and environmental. Presently, records show alcohol is the most abused drug in the U.S., and the problem is on the increase, especially among teenagers.

Researchers have established multiple nutrient deficiencies in those craving alcohol. Many are predisposed to alcoholism because of genetics. Those who have alcoholic parents or grandparents will have the same brain deficiencies which can lead to addictive behavior.

Dr. Roger Williams and his colleagues at the Clayton Foundation for Research at the University of Texas, established the vital research concerning the amino acid L-glutamine. Those craving alcohol have a definite glutamine deficiency. Dr. Williams and his associates observed that glutamine protects individuals against the poisonous effects of alcohol, and that it stops the craving for alcohol. They studied all the properties of glutamine and GABA, and found those who had addictive behaviors had deficiencies.

Glutamine and GABA decreases the craving for alcohol. Pure glutamine is tasteless, and can be mixed with food, water, or taken in capsule form. One alcoholic who was part of the study stopped drinking after he was given 3,000 mg of glutamine, daily, along with other necessary nutrients. Several studies demonstrated glutamine effectively reduces the craving for sweets. The same appetite center in the brain and hypothalamus protects against alcohol craving. Glutamine is the third most abundant amino acid in the blood and brain. Glutamine provides a major alternative fuel source when blood-sugar levels are low. Amino acids create the needed neurotransmitters to enhance the brain chemistry. A strong nutritional program is of utmost importance for the control of alcoholism and addictive behaviors.

For more information about alcohol addiction, read our book entitled, *Control Alcoholism with Amino Acids and Nutrients*. For prescribed addiction, read our updated book entitled, *Break Your Prescribed Addiction*.

Suggested Nutritional Support

The following program is for acute withdrawal and 3 months post sobriety. Continue with maintenance program outlined in our *Control Alcoholism* book after 3 months.

Glutamine powder or caps – 1,000 to 4,000 mg per day, divided. However, if you develop a craving for alcohol, open a capsule and pour directly onto your tongue to quickly stop the craving.

Rodex Forte (timed release) – 1 capsule per day that contains B6 (150 mg), B12 (200 mcg), and folic acid (800 mcg).

Mag Link – 4 to 6 tablets per day, divided OR

Mag Chlor 90, 15 to 25 drops, twice to four times daily, divided. If diarrhea or loose stools occur, take capsules or drops by spacing further apart or decrease dosage by 1.

Easy C (Esterified C) – 2 (500 mg) capsules, twice daily. If needed, add an additional 1000 mg of Easy C.

Tyrosine 850 – 1 (850 mg) twice per day for depression OR **DLPA 750 mg** – two, twice daily. **Caution:** *If you are taking an SSRI, SNRI, tricyclic, or MAOI antidepressant, or if you have a history of a melanoma, do not use Tyrosine.* **Caution:** *Do not use DLPA if you have PKU, pregnant, or lactating. Do not use tyrosine if you take MAO inhibitor or tricyclic antidepressants, or if you have a history of a melanoma.*

Decaf Green Tea Extract – 2 capsules, twice daily.

Mood Sync – 2 capsules, three time daily for anxiety and depression. **Caution:** *If you are taking an SSRI, SNRI, tricyclic, or MAOI antidepressant, or if you have a history of a melanoma, do not use Mood Sync.* Instead use Anxiety Control 2 capsules, three times daily, plus L–T,® 1 to 2 capsules, three times daily.

Anxiety Control 24 – 2 twice to three times per day, as needed, for stress and anxiety.

T-L Vite (multivitamin) – 1 capsule with noon meal.

Brain Link – 2 scoops in the morning and afternoon, depending on weight; if over 200 pounds, use 3 scoops OR use

SBNC – 2 capsules in the morning and afternoon.

ProDHA – 2 softgels, twice daily OR Pure Fish Oil Capsules – 1 softgel twice daily. **Caution:** *Do not use if you take anticoagulants (blood thinners), are allergic to iodine, or if you will have surgery within a week.*

Alpha Lipoic Acid – 1 (300 mg) capsules in the afternoon.

Sleep Link OR 5-HTP – 2 capsule (50 mg) an hour before bedtime, with juice. If needed, add 1 melatonin 3 mg capsule, or a 500 mg Mellow Mind (Ashwagandha). **Caution:** *If you are taking an SSRI, SNRI, tricyclic, or MAOI antidepressant, do not use Sleep Link or 5-HTP.* Instead use Anxiety Control, 2 capsules OR a 3 mg Melatonin capsule, 30 minutes before bed.

Neuro Links – dropperful as needed to reduce craving and calm your nerves during the acute withdrawal phase.

Liquid Serotonin – 10 to 12 drops, four times per day.

Adult A.D.D. / Hyperactivity

Recently, there has been an increase in the number of adults who feel they have ADD or ADHD, major problems they describe include their inability to concentrate, complete tasks, or stay focused. Many of them have turned to the powerful drug, Ritalin. Stimulant drugs such as Ritalin impair brain function and have no beneficial effect on the brain. According to Peter Breggin, M.D., in his book, *Talking Back to Ritalin,* Ritalin can either shrink or limit the growth of some areas of the brain, just as many psychiatric drugs can cause brain dysfunction and damage.

There are 16 adverse reactions listed in the *PDR (Physicians' Desk Reference)* for Ritalin. The most common adverse reactions are nervousness and insomnia. Other reactions include skin rashes, fever, anorexia, dizziness, palpitations, headaches, dyskinesia, drowsiness, blood pressure and pulse changes, pulse >100, angina, cardiac arrhythmias (heart rhythm disturbances), abdominal pain, and weight loss. Given this information, there should be no question about your decision.

Carefully providing sufficient amino acids supplies the brain and body what it needs to communicate and allows the brain to function at its peak. Amino acids must be supplied daily in adequate amounts for the brain to function properly. Simply stated, amino acids supply the fuel the brain requires to work properly.

Inadequate intake of ALA, EPA, and DHA (fish oils) or inability to metabolize EPA and DHA precursors contributes to ADHD according to researchers at Purdue University. Supplementing with EPA and DHA benefits ADHD patients. EFAs also affect mood and play a role in depression and other mood disorders.

There is no such thing as a Ritalin deficiency! There are many reasons why as we age our memory might not be what we feel it should be, but Ritalin is not the answer. Your brain cannot be deficient of Ritalin because it is never naturally present in your brain. If you cannot concentrate or stay focused, you need neurotransmitters. The following nutritional support program will help you nourish your brain so you feel better and think more clearly.

Suggested Nutritional Support

Brain Link Complex – Use per body weight; if over 200 pounds, 3 scoops in the morning OR

T–L Vite – 1 capsule daily (super multi-vitamin-mineral).

Glutamine – 2 (500 mg) capsules, twice daily or 1000 mg

of Super Glutamine Powder.

Mood Sync – 2 capsules in the morning, afternoon, and evening. **Caution:** *If you are taking an SSRI, SNRI, tricyclic, or MAOI antidepressant or if you have a history of a melanoma, do not use Mood Sync.*

Mag Link – 1 to 2 tablets, twice to three times daily OR **Mag Chlor 90** – 10 to 25 drops, twice to three times daily. *If diarrhea or loose stools occur, take capsules or drops by spacing further apart or decrease dosage by 1.*

ProDHA – 2 softgel, twice daily OR use **Pure Fish Oil** – 1 softgel, twice daily. **Caution:** *Do not use if you take anticoagulants (blood thinners) are allergic to iodine, or if you will have surgery within a week.*

5-HTP – 1 capsule, 30 minutes prior to bedtime. **Caution:** *If you take a SSRI, SNRI, tricyclic, or MAOI antidepressant, or if you have a history of a melanoma, do not use 5-HTP.*

Huperzine – 50 mcg capsule in the morning and in the evening. Huperzine derives from purified Chinese club moss and is a premier brain nutrient. Clinical studies confirm Huperzine enhances memory, and can be used by anyone twelve years of age or older. **Caution:** *Do not use if you are a pregnant or lactating woman, or if you have heart, pulmonary, or asthma problems.*

Phosphatidylserine (PS 100+) – 1 to 3 softgel(s) daily, divided. Phosphatidylserine (PS) is a phospholipid that is a component of brain cell membranes. Clinical studies demonstrate PS helps improve cognitive functions that decline with age including memory, learning, concentration, and vocabulary skills. Daily supplementation of PS provides more alertness and protects you against brain strain.

Neuro Links – 15 drops under the tongue to boost neurotransmitters in the brain. You should supplement with SBNC or Brain Link to boost your neurotransmitter levels.

Probiotics (Acidophilus) – Give some daily to boost good bacteria in the gut. Recent research shows a connection between the gut, the head, and behavior.

Special Note: If your symptoms become acute after

you eat certain foods, your problems could be related to food allergies. Millions of children and adults are diagnosed with ADD or ADHD when their problem is really food allergy related. For detailed information regarding ADD and ADHD, read our book, *Stop A.D.D. Naturally.*

Allergies / Sinus Problems

Allergies are the cause of sinus congestion and problems in about 90% of sinus cases. If you experience constant congestion and pressure, allergies could be the problem. Explore the possibility of chemical allergens as well as airborne. Food sensitivities/allergies can also cause congestion, stuffiness, headache, palpitations, upset stomach, fatigue, etc. If you eliminate or rotate the foods that contribute to your sinus problems, you help your body detoxify. Rotate your foods so you do not eat a particular food/food group any more frequently than every four to five days. For example, if you eat milk or milk products on Sunday, you would not eat any milk product in any form until Thursday or Friday. The time interval allows your body to recover from the exposure to the food you are sensitive to. So you feel better, have more energy, and have less problems with your allergies and sinuses. If certain foods continually cause problems, you may need to eliminate these foods from your diet.

Do not get hooked on nasal decongestant sprays such as Duration (Oxymetazoline). Nasal decongestants have a rebound effect requiring you to use them repeatedly. Instead use some saline (salt water) with MSM dissolved in distilled water to rinse your nose. Then use the homeopathic sprays.

You can make your own saline. In a glass container such as 4 cup measuring cup, combine 1 quart of distilled or purified water with 2 to 3 heaping teaspoons of pickling salt (Kosher salt) and 1 teaspoon of baking soda. Heat to boiling point, then allow to cool. Take care not to burn yourself. Store in sterile glass jar. The saline solution is good for 1 week. After the solution cools, use a bulb syringe or Nettie Pot to irrigate your sinuses. Irrigating your sinuses daily helps remove pollens and other irritants. For hypertonic saline, increase pickling salt to 4 teaspoons.

Allergies cause inflammation and congestion. By addressing inflammation, you battle congestion. Before NSAIDs (Non Steroidal Anti-Inflammatory Drugs) and steroids, doctors used enzymes and essentially fatty acids to reduce inflammation. Enzymes have an extremely wide safety range, and your body knows what to do with them.

Suggested Nutritional Support

NAC (N-Acetyl-Cysteine) – 1 600 mg capsule, twice to three times per day. NAC is a natural decongestant.

P5'P – 100 mg, morning and evening.

Tyrosine (500 mg) – 1 capsule in morning and 1 in evening. **Caution:** *If you take a SSRI, SNRI, tricyclic, or MAOI antidepressant, or if you have a history of a melanoma, do not use Tyrosine.*

Easy C (Esterified C) – 2,000 mg, three times per day.

Mag Link – 4 to 6 tablets per day, divided OR

Mag Chlor 90 – 15–25 drops in juice, 2 to 3 times daily. Magnesium helps prevent release of histamine. If diarrhea or loose stools occur, take tablets or drops by spacing further apart or decrease dosage by 1.

ProDHA – 2 softgels, twice to three times daily OR use

Pure Fish Oil Capsules – 2 softgels, twice daily. EFAs decrease inflammation and reduce allergic responses. **Caution:** *Do not use if you take anticoagulants (blood thinners) are allergic to iodine, or if you will have surgery within a week.*

Sea Buckthorn – 1 capsule twice daily. Sea Buckthorn

is a new super antioxidant that also has fatty acids. Sea Buckthorn has some anti-inflammatory properties that fights aging, and diseases associated with aging such heart disease, and cancer.

Heel Sinus (homeopathic) – 1 tablet every 15 minutes until improvement; then decrease to once every hour; then 1 tablet, four times per day.

Immune Health Basics (Beta Glucan) – 1 or 2 (75 mg) capsules, once or twice daily. Immune Health Basics activates and strengthens the immune system, and is about 200 times more powerful than echinacea. Use Immune Health Basics at intervals for an acute inflammatory or allergy reaction.

Decaf Green Tea Extract – 1 to 2 capsules, twice daily for antioxidant and anti-inflammatory properties.

PoweRelief – For headaches, use 1 or 2 capsules every 4 to 6 hours. Apply moist heat over your sinuses with your head elevated to promote sinus drainage. **Caution:** *Do not use if you have PKU. Do not use DLPA if you take MAO inhibitor or tricyclic antidepressants, pregnant, lactating, or if you have a history of a melanoma.*

MSM wash – Mix 1500 mg MSM in 2 ounces of distilled water. Using a bulb syringe, tilt your head to side and rinse each sinus.

Xlear Spray – Use spray as needed to moisturize and wash sinuses. Xlear contains a patented non-addictive wash designed for irritations caused by pollens and allergens. Xlear fights infections since 90% of all infection-causing bacteria in the sinuses and ears enters through the nose. Xlear contains xylitol, a naturally occurring sugar, that helps prevent bacteria from adhering to the cells in the nose or sinuses.

Sinusin Nasal Spray – Use as needed for nasal congestion. Sinusin helps normalize nasal tissues, and does not have a rebound effect.

Sinus & Allergy Nasal Spray (SAS) – 1 or 2 sprays into each nostril every four hours, or as needed. SAS is a natural homeopathic medicine without fear of histamine rebound. SAS provides temporary relief for symptoms associated with inflamed nasal passages such as sinus pressure and headache, congestion, runny nose, dry nasal passages, and sneezing. Use SAS year round for allergies due to respiratory allergies to pollen, animals, molds, yeast, or dust.

SerraEnzyme 80,000 I.U. – Use 1 to 3 capsules, 4 times daily divided for congestion, inflammation, or with a sinus infection. Sometimes antibiotics are necessary to combat a sinus infection.

Silver Nasal spray – 1 dropperful, two to four times daily as needed if you think you have or are getting a sinus infection.

Probiotics (Acidophilus) – Give some daily to boost good bacteria in the gut. Recent research shows a connection between the gut, the head, and behavior. Always use during and after a round of antibiotics.

Anti-Aging

Only you have the potential to change the way you live and age. Once you reach age 40, you hold the key to your productivity, your life-style, and the quality of your life. What is aging? Aging is breathing. Breathing oxygen produces free radicals that attack our cells! In effect, the very air you breathe in order to live, simultaneously causes you to age by rusting your body. In your teens and twenties, your cells were able to repair the damage caused by constant free radicals; but with age, oxygen attacks the body's mechanisms that replace and repair. With age, you become susceptible to damage from free radicals to your cell metabolism and your DNA. If you are over the age of 40, the damaging free radical process is now in place.

Once in the body, free radicals attack cell components and damage cells and tissues in the body. This free radical-induced damage alters the cell membrane structure and function. The membrane is no longer able to transport nutrients, oxygen, and water into the cell, and can no longer regulate the removal of waste products.

Free radicals also damage the cell's mitochondria, resulting in limited or halted production of energy for all cell processes. Free radical damage to enzymes and other proteins limits the body's building of tissues and causes accumulation of protein fragments. Both these conditions are recognized in premature aging of tissues. Finally, a cell cannot reproduce normally when free radicals alter the genetic code. Last resort: the cell dies, or the cell mutates to a cancerous cell.

Free radicals in the body are unavoidable. Your body produces free radicals as it processes food for energy. They form as a result of normal metabolic processes—during the formation of prostaglandins, or from normal intracellular oxygen metabolism. Free radicals are consumed in some foods, inhaled from air pollution and tobacco smoke, and generated in the environment from radiation and herbicides. Free radicals are thought be a factor in aging and certain diseases such as cardiovascular disease and cancer.

Fortunately, your body can use anti-free radical comprising antioxidants such as Vitamins C and E, beta-carotene, CoEnzyme Q10, NAC (N-Acetyl Cysteine), selenium, lutein, green tea, and glutathione. The Deluxe Scavenger contains most of these antioxidants. The recommended dose is 3 capsules, daily. Antioxidants protect the cells from free radical damage. In the *Psychopharmacology Journal* a study showed that Vitamin C reduced high cortisol levels from psychological stress. In this double blind study researchers gave 3000 mg of Vitamin C or a placebo to 120 volunteers. The volunteers were subjected to psychological stress to elevate cortisol levels by having to speak publically and

perform arithmetic tests. The volunteers th
Vitamin C had lower blood pressures, reported
stress and cortisol levels. Cortisol is a major stress
hormone produced by the adrenal glands. Elevations in
cortisol cause stress and aging in the body. Research
demonstrates that high cortisol levels may contribute to
degeneration and neuron death leading to loss of memory.
Control your stress so you control your cortisol level.
Sea Buckthorn is a newly discovered antioxidant. Sea
Buckthorn is a golden red fruit that provides essential
fatty acids including omega 7 as well as antioxidants rich
in glucosides, flavonoids, phenols, terpenes, vitamins E,
A, C, beta carotene, and trace elements. Sea Buckthorn
berries contain ten times more vitamin C than oranges,
and the third highest known source of Vitamin E in the
plant world.

Recent research suggests the antioxidants found in
tea, especially green tea, inhibit the growth of cancer and
may be a preventative for cancer due to the EGCGs or
catechins found in the tea. Green tea is one of the best all
round antioxidant scavengers known to man and tea has
been consumed for over 5,000 years in China and India.

As the aging process progresses, other physiological
changes take place, including increased fat levels and decreased muscle mass. Additionally, you have decreased
bone mass, decreased water intake and content, and increased fatigue. No two people age the same, so the exact point at which decline begins is different for everyone. The majority of gerontologists agree that 50 seems
to be the magic number.

The key to controlling the aging process is to assist
the brain and body to recreate homeostasis of youth.
How do you do this? By supplying needed nutrients
such as growth hormone, the connecting link between
the brain and body. Scientists have found that amino
acids will induce growth hormone secretion. The amino

acid, glutamine, is most used by the body during times of stress, anxiety, depression, grief, and chronic pain. Your immune system and gut live on glutamine. If your body does not produce enough glutamine, you will experience memory and focus problems, muscle loss, as well as immune dysfunction. Your gut will atrophy, keeping valuable nutrients from being absorbed.

According to Dr. Ronald Klatz, President of the Academy of Anti-Aging Medicine, and author of *Grow Young with HGH,* glutamine is an effective growth hormone releaser that crosses the blood-brain barrier where it increases energy and mental alertness. People with low glutamine levels have higher rates of arthritis, diabetes, and heart disease; those with high glutamine levels feel and perform much better. The recommended dose is 2 grams of glutamine powder at bedtime and an additional gram may be used in the morning for a jumpstart. Glutamine is an inhibitory neurotransmitter vital in smooth brain function.

DHEA, a neurohormone produced primarily by the adrenal cortex, is the most abundant steroid hormone in humans. In his book, *DHEA, The Youth Hormone,*

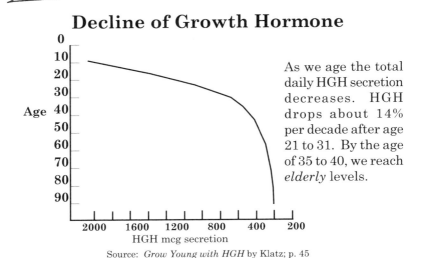

Decline of Growth Hormone

As we age the total daily HGH secretion decreases. HGH drops about 14% per decade after age 21 to 31. By the age of 35 to 40, we reach *elderly* levels.

Source: *Grow Young with HGH* by Klatz; p. 45

C. Norman Shealy, M.D., reports DHEA deficiencies in all patients with major diseases, including those with obesity, diabetes, high blood pressure, cancer, various immune deficiencies, coronary artery disease, and autoimmune disorders. Chronic stress syndrome uses available DHEA in the brain in concentrations equal to those in the adrenal cortex. Dr. Shealy's research "established the most important metabolic effects of DHEA: it stabilizes glucose, regulates all other hormones, decreases cholesterol, acts as a precursor to estrogen and testosterone, assists homeostasis due to chronic stress, enhances immune function, maintains youth and health, and stabilizes weight." DHEA should not be used until after the age of 40, unless blood tests verify your DHEA level to be low. The recommended dosage is to start with 25 mg, upon awakening in the morning; if you are over the age of 50 or weigh over 200 pounds, start with 50 mg. The best way to establish your needs is to have your blood tested for DHEA sulfate level. This will tell you exactly what your body needs. Most major labs can do this test.

Research demonstrates the importance of DHA and EPA (essential fatty acids or EFAs). EFAs, linoleic acid (LA) and Alpha Linolenic Acids (ALA) are the major building blocks of fat in the body. These fats are essential because the body cannot manufacture them. Since 70% of all deaths in the U.S. relate to deficiencies, excesses, or imbalances of fat, Americans do not consume enough good fat. The importance of EFAs include maintenance of cell membranes, development and function of brain and nerve tissues, oxygen transfer and energy production, immune support, local hormones, and inflammatory responses. EFAs play a part with moods and mood disorders. EFAs play a role in the cardiovascular system, especially atherosclerosis and stroke, asthma and allergies, cancer, brain function, immune system, joints, and even your eyes. In the *American Journal of Clinical Nutrition*, researchers from the Brigham and Women's Hospital in

Boston found that the higher the consumption of omega-3 rich foods such as tuna fish, the less cases of dry eye syndrome were seen.

In June 2003 a study published in *Diabetes Management* gave seven volunteers 7.2 grams of fish oil per day for three weeks. They were exposed to mental stress tests that increased blood pressure, heart rate, and cortisol levels. After three weeks of the fish oil supplementation, the increase in cortisol levels was greatly reduced when stress tested. In the 2004 issue of *Stress* a study looked at the effects of phophatidylserine on endocrine and psychological responses to mental stress. This double blind study consisting of 40 men and 40 women, aged 20 to 45, subjected these subjects to mental arthrimetic challenges. These volunteers received either 400 mg, 600 mg, or a placebo daily before the arthrimetic challenge. Phosphatidylserine effectively reduced the cortisol response to the subjects that received 400 mg, and the subjects that received 600 mg showed a significant reduction in cortisol levels. Phosphatidylserine helps to reduce stress effects on the body and slows aging.

Since fish are at the bottom of the food chain, their tissues contain higher amounts of mercury and pesticides. Heavy metals and pesticides pose problems for possible damage to the body. In this case, supplementing with purified fish oils may be a healthier alternative along with some Vitamin E.

As we age, our ability to digest food decreases, as the enzymes needed to digest foods are not produced in the quantity necessary and enzyme activity diminishes greatly. Efficient digestion only takes place if there is an adequate amount of enzymes. Enzymes are essential to life and the human body cannot function without enzymes. Enzymes are necessary for food digestion and absorption, strong immune system, and body movement (muscles). Enzymes help the body utilize amino acids and facilitate their functions.

Stress affects the digestive system by reducing the amount of digestive juices and diverting blood away from digestive muscles to other muscles in the body. Anxieties, agitation, worry, or fatigue can lead to disturbances in the gastrointestinal (GI) tract interfering with digestion and nutrient absorption.

In *Survival Into the 21st Century,* Viktor Kulvinskas states the physiological symptoms of long-term indigestion are numerous including: the lips become puffy and pouty, producing a sad look, the irises change color becoming darker and cloudier, a crease develops in the middle of the tongue, and bags develop under the eyes (a sign of kidney and adrenal stress). Other symptoms include bad breath, heartburn, belching, burping, flatulence, slow stomach emptying time, abdominal bloating, constipation and/or diarrhea, skin problems, reoccurring headaches, mental fatigue, lack of energy and vitality, difficulty concentrating, and food allergies. In the *Secret of Life* by James B. Sumner, he states that people over 40 often feel old due to reduced enzyme levels in the body.

Clinical studies show that most digestive problems are due to pancreatic enzyme insufficiency. The pancreas is stressed, overworked, and then problems begin to occur. Pancreatin is a digestive enzyme that helps breakdown foods (proteins, fats, and carbohydrates) for absorption into the body. Pancreatin is a vital enzyme produced by the pancreas. Enzymes are the keys to proper digestion and improve overall health. You need protease (proteins), amylase (carbohydrates), and lipase (fats) enzymes to digest foods. A good source of these enzymes is pancreatin. You will notice how much better you feel.

Other Anti-Aging Nutritional Support

CoEnzyme Q10 – 30 to 150 mg, per day. CoEnzyme Q10 helps support the immune system, heart, and helps control the flow of oxygen within the cells.

Easy C (Esterified C)– 2,000 to 3,000 mg, divided. Easy C is an antioxidant that supports your immune system while lowering your cortisol levels (stress hormone released by your adrenals).

Vitamin E – 800 I.U., per day. Vitamin E is an antioxidant that helps retard aging and helps protect the heart and blood vessels.

Huperzine A – 1 (50 mcg) capsule in the morning, for memory and mind enhancement. Huperzine derives from purified Chinese club moss. Clinical studies confirm Huperzine enhances memory. Huperzine was featured in the *Journal of American Medical Association (JAMA)*, and is recommended by neurologists. **Caution:** *Do not use Huperzine if you are a pregnant or lactating woman, or if you have congestive heart failure, hypertension (high blood pressure) or pulmonary problems.*

Brain Link Complex – 2 to 3 scoops, twice daily in the morning and afternoon.

Green Tea Extract (Decaf) – 1 to 2 (500 mg) capsules, twice daily.

ProDHA – 2 softgels, twice daily OR

Pure Fish Oil Capsules – 1 softgel, twice daily (EFAs). More than 60% of the human brain is composed of fat, especially an omega-3 fatty acid called docosahexaenoic acid (DHA). DHA is needed for optimal signal transmissions in the brain, nervous system, and the eye, and is essential in the diet. Foods such as fish and egg yolks are rich sources of DHA. **Caution:** *Do not use if you take anticoagulants (blood thinners), are allergic to iodine, or if you will have surgery within a week.*

Flax – 1 heaping teaspoon, twice daily, dissolved in juice or sprinkled over a food such as salad. Fortified flax is a rich source of omega 3, plus it provides fiber to help alleviate constipation and keep your intestines healthy.

Digestive enzymes (such as Super Pancreatin 650) – 1 to 2 capsules with each meal. As we age, we do not replace the enzymes used to digest foods; so our enzyme levels decrease in the body.

Mag Link – 4 to 6 tablets per day, divided OR

Mag Chlor 90 – 15–25 drops in juice, 2 to 3 times daily. Magnesium helps prevent release of histamine. *If diarrhea or loose stools occur, take tablets or drops by spacing further apart or decrease dosage by 1.* Mag Link and Mag Chlor provides magnesium chloride, the same form of magnesium present in the body, so it is readily absorbed and tolerated.

Cal, Mag, Zinc Complex – 4 capsules, at bedtime.

Melatonin – 1 (3 mg) capsule, 30 minutes to an hour prior to bedtime. *Use melatonin only if you are over 30 years of age.* Melatonin helps promote sleep and is a powerful antioxidant.

DHEA – 25 to 50 mg daily upon awakening on an empty stomach.

Pregnenolone – 10 to 50 mg daily, upon awakening in the morning. Pregnenolone is a direct precursor to DHEA and progesterone, and serves as the building block for all other steroid hormones. When the pregnenolone level drops, usually when you reach the age of 30, it negatively affects your mental function, memory, mood, and energy levels.

NAC (N-Acetyl Cysteine) – 1 capsule, twice daily. NAC is a precursor to glutathione, an antioxidant, and natural decongestant. Glutathione protects the body against natural and man-made oxidants.

Colon Balance – for IBS problems, 1 capsule, three times daily. See IBS section, pages 179–180.

Other Factors

Exercise for 30 to 45 minutes at least 4 times per week. Exercise reduces your stress and your cortisol levels. Start very slowly and gradually increase. Walking is one of the best all round exercises. If you have not exercised in the last year, it is best to have a checkup with your doctor and get his clearance.

Meditation helps reduce your stress levels.

Eat 4 to 5 servings of fruits and vegetables a day along with whole grain and nuts. Use organic fruits and vegetables to avoid pesticides that may alter your cells over time. Remember, pesticides are stored in your fat and may remain there forever.

Probiotics (Acidophilus) – Eat some yogurt, kefir milk, or take a good acidophilus supplement daily. Recent research shows a connections between the gut, the head, and behavior. Probiotics help keep a balance in your gut, fighting yeast and other organisms that would like to live in such a cozy spot. The gut is the perfect environment so yeast grow rampantly if not controlled by the good bacteria in your intestines.

Brain Boosters
Memory and Concentration

The brain is the busiest, yet the most undernourished organ in the body. The brain is the master controller, the programmer for every movement, mood, breath, heartbeat, thought, even for body temperature and hormone balance. Our brain uses 20% of the body's total energy supply, so energy must be supplied on a constant basis in the form of nutrition and nutrients. Oxygen and glucose are in constant demand as fuel by the brain. The brain uses 25% of the body's total oxygen intake. Blood carries these nutrients to the brain at a rate of 1½ pints per minute. The brain uses oxygen and glucose first, then protein, fat, amino acids, vitamins, and minerals. Fats (lipids) make up 50 to 60% of structural brain matter, but amino acids provide the neurotransmitters your brain needs to communicate. Research has demonstrated that poor nutrition at any time in our life can permanently alter brain development.

Your state of nutrition equals the state of your brain's health and functioning. How your brain functions depends on how you nourish your mind and body, especially in today's stressful world. Stress and anxiety severely deter proper brain function. The quality of brain function depends on neurotransmitters, the chemical language of the brain. Neurotransmitters carry impulses from one neuron to another, as from one cell to another cell, such as a muscle cell. Neurotransmitters can either be inhibitory or excitatory. The balance determines whether motor neurons fire. If stress, anxiety, depression, or chronic pain cause major deficiencies, irregular firing can occur. Irregular firing of motor neurons sends mixed messages to the brain and can cause you to display maladaptive behavior.

Since 1975, scientists have identified more than fifty neurotransmitters, but the communications conducted between brain cells use only approximately ten major neurotransmitters. The best known neurotransmitters are serotonin, epinephrine, norepinephrine, and acetylcholine. Serotonin comes from the precursor amino acid tryptophan, or 5-HTP. Epinephrine synthesizes from the amino acid phenylalanine, or tyrosine. Acetylcholine metabolizes from the B complex substance known as choline.

The following nutrients are important for proper brain function.

SBNC (Super Balanced Neurotransmitter Complex®) helps maintain a balance of amino acids in the brain. SBNC contains a balance of the amino acids glutamine, GABA, taurine, phenylalanine, glycine, arginine, methionine, leucine, valine, lysine, isoleucine, alanine, and histidine. Pyridoxal 5' Phosphate (B6), acts as an activating agent. Either children or adults can use this formula.

Glutamine was established as the memory and concentration amino acid by University of Texas premier researcher Dr. Roger Williams. Glutamine is found in the nerves of the hippocampus—the memory center of the brain, in the cranial nerves, and in numerous receptors throughout the brain and body. As the third most abundant amino acid in the blood and brain, glutamine helps the brain dispose of waste ammonia, a protein breakdown by-product. Glutamine provides a major alternative fuel source for the brain with low blood-sugar levels. Ginkgo Biloba, a brain booster herb, has an excellent track record for enhancing memory and concentration. Ginkgo increases blood flow to the head, and improves mental functioning and the ability to focus for longer periods of time. Senior citizens report excellent results combining Ginkgo and Glutamine. Ginkgo may increase bleeding in surgery. If you are having surgery, stop using ginkgo at least 36 hours prior to surgery, preferably a week before.

Researchers at Purdue University report insufficient intake of ALA, EPA, and DHA (fish oils) or the inability to metabolize EPA and DHA precursors contribute to ADHD. These researchers concluded that supplementation was beneficial for ADHD patients. Deficiencies of EFAs are found in patients with Alzheimer's, other dementias, and in cognitive impairment with aging. Low serum DHA levels are also seen with depression. Brain fatty acids are replaced at 2 to 8% per day for DHA and 3 to 5% for AA (arachonic acid).

Huperzine serrata, or Chinese club moss, comes from the mountains of China and has been used for centuries to improve memory, focus, and concentration, and to help alleviate memory problems among the elderly. Research data indicates an estimated 100,000 people have been successfully treated. Huperzine is safe and effective as reported in the *Journal of the American Medical Association*. Huperzine, a natural, potent, and selective cholinesterase inhibitor proves superior to other acetylcholinesterase inhibitors. Scientific research demonstrates multiple therapeutic benefits of Huperzine use in the following areas: learning and memory retention, improved focus and concentration, treatment of cognitive and memory impairment, and improved nerve transmission signals to muscles. Huperzine A has been very effective for those suffering from Alzheimer's disease.

Alzheimer's patients go through a progressive loss of neuron groups that inhibits communication in the brain and causes destruction of the cerebral cortex, the outer tissue of the brain. A major characteristic of Alzheimer's and progressive loss of mental cognitive function is oxidative stress that increases the rate at which the disease progresses. **Note:** *If you have a problem with heart or pulmonary disease, or if you are pregnant or lactating, you should not use Huperzine.*

Oxidative stress results from free radical damage. Brain cells are very susceptible to oxidative stress. To protect the brain from oxidative stress, you must take antioxidants on a daily basis. The Deluxe Scavengers formula contains the antioxidants, CoQ10, Beta-Carotene, Vitamins C and E, riboflavin, lemon bioflavonoids, Selenium, Glutathione, NAC, and B6, all in one capsule.

Minerals prove vital to brain function, and magnesium, as well as acting as a major cofactor for all amino acids, ensures smooth muscle function. You have 657 muscles in your body that require magnesium every second of every day. The best source of magnesium is Mag Link, magnesium chloride, the same form of magnesium that naturally occurs in your cells.

Phosphatidylserine (PS) revitalizes cognitive functions that decline with age—memory, learning, concentration, even vocabulary skills. Extremely well documented, PS has been researched in more than 60 human clinical studies over a period of more than 20 years, in both North America and Europe. Seventeen double-blind, controlled, clinical trials prove, beyond doubt, the considerable worth of PS as a dietary supplement. These consistently positive clinical findings, backed by more than 2,800 scientific research papers, prove that PS safely and effectively supports memory, learning, concentration, word recall, and a wide range of other cognitive brain functions.

Besides benefiting cognition, PS benefits other brain

activities, like coping with stress, fighting depression, and maintaining daily hormone rhythms. In young, healthy men, PS lowered the production of stress hormones linked to strenuous exercise, and eased stress-related mood symptoms in the elderly. Phosphatidylserine enriches all our brain cells, which helps them produce and release the natural chemical transmitters that make the brain work.

But, while drugs can be used to raise or lower the levels of single chemical transmitters, PS influences many major transmitter systems to produce an overall harmonizing influence on the brain. Phosphatidylserine also helps the brain process energy. The brain requires a lot of energy to carry out its function. The membranes of the mitochondria—the energy powerhouses of the nerve cells—carry out the vast majority of the cell energy functions. PS gets into these membranes, alongside Coenzyme Q10 and Vitamin E, improving energy efficiency.

For those who require all their vitamins, minerals, and amino acids in one complex, Brain Link, a complete neurotransmitter complex, supplies the body and brain with all the needed nutrients. Brain Link proves excellent for children, or adults, and can be mixed with any fruit juice. Brain Link is especially effective for those who have absorption problems and require a faster breakdown of nutrients.

Pregnenolone, the super hormone for your brain, enhances memory, improves concentration, and fights mental fatigue. Pregnenolone is one key to keeping your brain functioning at peak capacity even into your 80s. Some scientists believe it is the most potent memory enhancer of all time. Pregnenolone is produced in the brain and in the adrenal cortex, the gland that sits above the kidneys. Pregnenolone production declines with age. By the time you reach 75, you produce 60% less pregnenolone than you did in your 30s. Super hormones, like pregnenolone, are similar to neurotransmitters. Located in the brain, they have a profound impact on mental function. Pregnenolone works with the amino acid GABA to enhance brain function. Clinical studies demonstrate that those with low levels of pregnenolone have clinical depression, as well as memory and concentration problems.

Galantamine derives from a plant called Galanthus nivalis. Galantamine is a neuro nutrient that enhances cholinergic neurotransmission from an increase in acetylcholine levels in prefrontal cortex. Secondly, it offers neuroprotection by increasing the release of acetylcholine. A new discovery with Galantamine is its ability to dismantle beta-amyloid through A phagocytosis (white blood cells that engulf and digest microorganisms and cellular debris). This is on the cutting edge with long-term cognitive benefits for Alzheimer's patients.

Vinpocetine is potent antioxidant that derives from periwinkle plant, Vinca Minor. Vinpocetine supports brain metabolism by elevating cerebral synthesis of ATP (cell energy). Clinical studies show that Vinpocetine increases blood flow to the brain thereby increasing more oxygen to the brain. Enhanced circulation increases the concentration of neurotransmitters such as acetylcholine, serotonin, dopamine, and norepinephrine that supports better cognition and memory, attention, and normal brain functions.

The brain is a super computer—but a computer must have constant nourishment to continue to produce the data we need, from childhood to our golden years.

Suggested Nutritional Support

SBNC – 1 or 2 capsules in the morning and afternoon. SBNC provides needed neurotransmitters to improve memory and concentration.

Brain Link – 2 to 3 scoops, in the morning and in the afternoon, depending on weight.

Glutamine Powder (1000 mg per scoop) – 1 scoop, twice

daily, in water or juice OR

Glutamine capsules (500 mg) – 2 capsules, twice to three times daily.

ProDHA – 2 softgels, twice to three daily OR use

Pure Fish Oil Capsules – 1 softgels, twice to three times daily, divided (EFAs). **Caution:** *Do not use if you take anticoagulants (blood thinners), are allergic to iodine, or if you will have surgery within a week.*

Huperzine A – 1 capsule, twice daily. **Caution:** *Do not use Huperzine if pulmonary problems or Congestive Heart Failure exist, or if you are pregnant or lactating.*

Ginkgo – 1 (40 mg) capsule, twice daily. **Caution:** *If you are taking anticoagulants (blood thinners), have a bleeding disorder, or have surgery or dental procedures, do not use Ginkgo.* If in doubt, talk with your health care practitioners.

Pregnenolone (PG) – 10 to 50 mg daily, depending on your age, upon awakening in morning. PG is a direct precursor of DHEA. Dr. Regelson calls PG the most potent memory enhancer available.

Deluxe Scavengers – 3 capsules, daily.

T-L Vite – 1 capsule, daily, with main meal. This formulation contains, in one capsule, all the vitamins needed for better brain function.

Mag Link – 4 to 6 tablets per day, divided OR

Mag Chlor 90 – 15–25 drops in juice, 2 to 3 times daily. *If diarrhea or loose stools occur, take tablets or drops by spacing further apart or decrease dosage by 1.*

Phosphatidylserine (PS 100+) – 1 (100 mg) softgel, one to three times daily, divided.

Green Tea Extract (Decaf) – 1 capsule twice daily.

Galantamine (GalantaMind) – for Alzheimer's like symptoms, add 4 mg daily for a week. After 1 week, add a second 4 mg capsule. If desired, after another week, add a third or total of 12 mg per day. Take with food. Galantamine can cause some nausea symptoms.

Vinpocetine – 10 mg, three times a day.

Carpal Tunnel Syndrome
Repetitive Stress Injury

Carpal tunnel syndrome (CTS) is a neuropathy caused by an entrapment and compression of the medial nerves as they pass through the carpal tunnel area of the wrist. This results in a loss of motor function, including pain, numbness, and tingling in the middle three fingers. Other clinical symptoms include a pins-and-needle sensation in the entire hand, sleep disturbances, and weakness progressing to atrophy centered around the hand and wrist. Warning signs include pain, numbness, a tingling or burning sensation, weakness or loss of grip strength, and loss of sleep due to discomfort.

Repetitive stress/strain injuries (RSI) have now become known as the workplace curse of the new millennium. RSI symptoms can include everything from neck and shoulder pain, to back strain, all caused by prolonged repetitive movements involved in certain occupations or recreational activities. Manual tasks that repeatedly flex and extend the wrist intensify CTS with swelling and by compressing the wrist nerves. RSI may hit abruptly or have a slow onset involving one or both hands. The nerves must receive proper nourishment, or the symptoms caused by the lack of nourishment cause the median nerve to short circuit, requiring you to seek treatment. Do not delay treatment; your thumb, index finger, and middle finger can atrophy the thenar (palm) muscle, rendering your hand permanently useless.

The standard medical treatments for CTS include cortisone injections and surgery to relieve the pressure on the nerve. Sometimes these treatments cause permanent disabilities, in addition to the consequences of failing to address a B6 deficiency. In one twelve week study, twenty-two patients with CTS were given between 50 to 300 mg of B6. All but one of the thirty-nine affected hands responded to the B6 treatment—a 97.4% cure rate!

B6 works by correcting the function of the synovium, the sheath encompassing the tendons. B6 stimulates the body's production of cortisone, thus decreasing the swelling in the tendon sheath, which, in turn, releases the pressure on the median nerve. Hyaluronic acid, the lubricant inside joints and the carpal tunnel, needs B6 to be produced by the body.

Suggested Nutritional Support

Rodex Forte – 1 timed-release capsule daily that contains B6 (150 mg), B12 (200 mcg), and folic acid (800 mcg).

DMSO – Apply topically to wrist, as needed, for swelling.

Mag Link – 2 tablets, twice daily for muscle tension OR **Mag Chlor 90** – 15–25 drops in juice, 2 to 3 times daily. *If diarrhea or loose stools occur, take tablets or drops by spacing further apart or decrease dosage by 1.*

Glucosamine & Chondroitin – 500 mg capsule Glucosamine along with 400 mg Chondroitin, three times daily.

PoweRelief – 1 or 2 capsules, every 6 hours, as needed for pain. **Caution:** *Do not use PoweRelief if you have PKU, take a MAO inhibitor or tricyclic antidepressants, or if you have a history of a melanoma.* Apply **Mag MAXX** topically to the wrist, twice daily.

SerraEnzyme 80,000 I.U. – 1 to 3 capsules, twice to three times daily, to support tissue repair, reduce swelling, inflammation, and pain.

Easy C (Esterified C) – 1,000 mg, morning and evening.

Magnetic wrist tube or wrap support – wear daily, as needed.

Mood Sync – 1 capsule, twice daily, for mood support. **Caution:** *Do not use if you are taking an SSRI, SNRI, tricyclic, or MAOI antidepressant, or have had a melanoma.*

Ice Pack – At night, use an ice pack to reduce swelling and pain.

ProDHA – 2 softgels, twice daily OR

Pure Fish Oil Capsules – 1 capsules, twice daily to enhance the production of anti-inflammatory eicosanoids, and reduce the production of pro-inflammatory eicosanoids. **Caution:** *Do not use if you take anticoagulants (blood thinners), are allergic to iodine, or if you will have surgery within a week.*
MSM – 750 mg, three times daily. MSM is a dry form of DMSO, dimethyl sulfoxide, a naturally occurring sulfur compound and nutrient. MSM reduces pain, improves blood supply, and lowers muscle spasms and inflammation involved in CTS.

Chronic Emotional Fatigue

Millions of people suffer from Chronic Emotional Fatigue (CEF) and Chronic Stress Syndrome (CSS). The complexities of these pervasive problems indicate the need for more extensive research, information, and patient education. CEF and Stress Syndrome are not psychiatric problems and cannot be addressed by treating with antidepressants, tranquilizers, or pain pills.

Because of the complex natures of chronic emotional fatigue and chronic stress syndrome, patients must understand how their brain and body store emotions. Emotions are simultaneously everywhere in the body. Emotion-and stress-related thoughts always move in an upward direction, which increases or causes anxiety after an emotional experience.

Chronic emotional fatigue and stress syndrome do not happen overnight. They accumulate over months or years from non-stop fatigue and stress exhaustion. The program outlined in this text helps you heal and gives you a key to unlock the door that leads you to health, happiness, and peace of mind. You must take one day at a time and be patient with yourself or with a loved one

Symptoms of Chronic Emotional Fatigue and Chronic Stress Syndrome

1. Anxiety
2. Mood swings
3. Mental and physical fatigue
4. Sluggishness
5. Chronic muscle spasms
6. Uncertainty
7. Fear that comes and goes
8. Panic attacks
9. Sleep problems
10. Chronic digestive upset
11. Constant body aches and pains
12. Stiff neck and/or limited range of motion
13. Muscle jerks
14. Churning stomach
15. Eye strain
16. Loss of interest (in everything)
17. No sex drive
18. Pounding heart, skipped beats
19. Low self esteem
20. No confidence
21. Withdrawal
22. Sensitivity to bright lights
23. Sensitivity to noise, especially loud sounds
24. Depression
25. Tension headaches or other headaches
26. Constant stress
27. Blurred vision
28. Constant fear of failure
29. Feelings of helplessness and hopelessness
30. Feelings of guilt
31. As fatigued in the morning, upon awakening, as when you went to bed.
32. Apathy
33. Tension

who is suffering.

Chronic emotional fatigue and chronic stress syndrome bring about an intense, painful, nagging loss of control that affects every nerve fiber in your brain and body. Few people recognize it or know that the many symptoms they dread are no more than the symptoms of constant, unrelenting chronic stress that leads to full-blown emotional fatigue. However, the knowledge and understanding of what is happening to you is a very powerful healer.

For more than twenty years, I have watched patients go from doctor to doctor, looking for a magic bullet they never find. A magic bullet does not exist. Chronic emotional fatigue can attack you as physical fatigue, or emotional fatigue. This constant feeling of anxiety, or mental fatigue, keeps you from being able to function on a daily basis. Emotional fatigue uses nervous energy and allows the chemicals produced by muscular fatigue, such as lactic acid, to collect throughout the body. This is one reason why anxious people often complain of aching legs, back, necks, and even arms. This kind of ache is so intense that standing for short periods of time causes very anxious or stressed people to look for some type of support to lean on, or to head straight home to bed. When pain and fatigue consume your body day and night, you lose the will to get better.

Stress causes chronic fatigue and chronic stress syndrome. Stress-induced illness is an accumulation of psychological and physical stress responses throughout your life. Emotional fatigue and chronic stress, in part, come from home or work. You are also influenced by your toxic environment, negative information, violence, crowded expressways, traumatic events, disease, or anything that makes you feel a loss of control over your life. Taking care of a loved one who is terminally ill, then experiencing the death, leaves you helpless, hopeless, and with feelings that consume your days and nights. Sometimes you even take on the same symptoms as the loved one you lost—even the same pain—but you have NO disease. What you feel is psychosomatic in nature: there is no pathology or disease. This does not mean there is no pain or fatigue. In fact, your body is overwhelmed with it. The longer you experience uncertainty, fear, stress, and anxiety, the more saturated your mind becomes. Mental stress then turns into physical symptoms.

Many patients in mid life tell me they begin to recall traumatic experiences from their childhood. This is not unusual when emotional fatigue controls your life. Each time you felt loss of control in your life experiences, it left an imprint on your brain. These experiences will resurface because they've been stored in your memory as negative, repressed emotions. Repressed emotions and stress are stored in every cell and every muscle of your body. This, alone, can cause symptoms of emotional fatigue, depression, and pain. Many sufferers live in their doctor's offices, having one test after another. They are ready and want to believe something is physically wrong with them. An actual illness would prevent their having to face the stress of dealing with and resolving their repressed negative experiences. When you live in the past, you are consumed by the past. When the past intrudes on the present, it brings forth a very powerful force of pain, emotional fatigue, and depression. For healing to occur, you must deal with all your feelings as they occur. Then you can let them go instead of recording them for later playback and more suffering.

Emotional fatigue and depression go hand in hand, because depression depletes the mind and body. Depression implies a downward direction, a depth out of which a depressed person must somehow drag him-or-herself. Most feel it as an endless struggle, but it does not have to be such. Do not struggle to lift yourself out of anything. Direct your energy to clearing yourself, not only from negative, depleting depression, but from chronic fatigue. Stop struggling and start healing.

Rushing around, trying to get yourself out of depression can increase your fatigue and depletion. Going out, meeting people, and keeping busy help. Too often, you feel better when you are out, but become depressed as soon as you see your home. You begin playing old tapes or recordings in your mind.

Please remember, recovery from depletion is gradual. You dipped deeply into your emotional reserves. It will take time for these reserves to be replenished, just as a wound takes time to heal. This means you must work with your feelings of depression. You must be prepared to take them with you, even though they press heavily on your heart, and you feel a load of lead in your lungs.

If your doctor suggests antidepressants, they are not the answer; they will not help. Tell your doctor you prefer using a natural alternative such as amino acids. Amino acids treat the problem, not just the symptoms. Orthomolecular therapists and doctors know how to treat chronic emotional fatigue. You must restore your immune system and balance your brain chemistry.

If you are willing to work on understanding that feelings of depression are a form of depletion, the temporary symptoms soon pass. Time and healing gradually recharge your batteries, especially after the age of forty. Do not be impatient!

Constant, anxious inward thinking in chronic emotional fatigue brings *brain drain*—mental fatigue. Thoughts slow down and thinking becomes an effort. In a chronically, emotionally drained person, thoughts come with a great deal of effort. It is almost as if each thought has to be worked through twice. These sufferers become easily confused, finding concentration and remembering arduous.

When mental fatigue and sensitization work together,

they throw off frightening ideas that seem impossible. Do not let this disturb you, and don't use your energy fighting unwanted thoughts. Just let them flow so you can work to either resolve or let them go. If you fight them, you add more tension and make the thoughts seem even more important. What you make important is more difficult to forget. Do not fight to forget them, just tell yourself they are unimportant. See them for what they are—only thoughts. Work with them and, with time, they will dissolve.

Fatigue accentuates unreality. Fatigue of the eye muscles interferes with the functioning of the lens. Vision seems blurred, so you have difficulty focusing. You notice it more when looking from a near object to a distant one, or vice versa. Objects in bright sunlight seem as if they are in dark shadows. The sufferer complains that everything suddenly goes dark, provoking fear. But, these symptoms are only temporary. Because you do not understand that this black world is caused by eye-muscle fatigue, you panic. You add more stress and tension to your body, so it takes longer for the world to return to its normal brightness.

Can you see how important it is to understand the chronic fatigue progression? Most people do not know how fear and fatigue trick you into thinking the wrong things. Again, acceptance, staying in reality, letting your mind and body float, drift, and relax are the keys!

In many ways, suffering like yours is a marker. We learn by contrast. Until we know emotional pain, we never know the true meaning of peace, and God knows you have known pain. Later, when you are able to step back and look at your life, things take on a new meaning. The pain is not as intense, and you are able to understand physical and mental fatigue. Never regret what you have been through. Your journey was a learning experience. Starting now, this very moment—not tomorrow—try your best to accept it. Stop struggling and fighting the rain.

When you stop the struggle, you gradually return to your old self but with more understanding and sensitivity. Your energy will come back, and you will, again, look forward to each day of life.

Chronic emotional fatigue attacks those who cannot express, sort out, or deal with stress, anxiety, depression, fear, or grief. Do not repress. Express. If someone is trying to take control of your life, declare yourself! You take control of your life. Use health, happiness, and peace of mind as the keys to the best quality of life you've ever dreamed possible! For more help, read my book, *Post Trauma and Chronic Emotional Fatigue.*

Suggested Nutritional Support

DHEA – Upon arising, take 1 (25 mg) capsule, if over 40; 1 (50 mg) capsule, if over 60.

Brain Link Complex – 3 scoops daily in the mornings OR **T-L Vite** – 1 capsule with 2 Super Balanced Neurotransmitter Complex (SBNC) capsules.

Deluxe Scavenger – 3 capsules, daily.

CoEnzyme Q10 – 50 mg to 100 mg daily.

Mag Link – 2 tablets, twice to three times daily OR **Mag Chlor 90** – 15–25 drops in juice, 2 to 3 times daily. *If diarrhea or loose stools occur, take tablets or drops by spacing further apart or decrease dosage by 1.*

Mood Sync – 2 capsules, three times per day. If you feel more anxiety, add an Anxiety Control capsule in place of 1 Mood Sync. **Caution:** *Do not use if you are taking an SSRI, SNRI, tricyclic, or MAOI antidepressant, or have had a melanoma.*

Digestive enzyme or **Super Pancreatin 650** – 2 with each meal.

Easy C (Esterified C) – 2 (500 mg) capsules in the morning and in the evening.

Alpha KG – 1 capsule, three times daily.

Chromium Picolinate – 1 (200 mcg) capsule.

5-HTP – 1 (50 mg) capsule, 1 hour prior to bedtime.

Caution: *If you are taking an SSRI, or SNRI, tricyclic, or MAOI antidepressant, do not use 5-HTP.*

Probiotics (Acidophilus) – Give some daily to boost good bacteria in the gut. Recent research shows a connections between the gut, the head, and behavior.

Use the following supplements as needed.

Chronic pain – 2 capsules of **PoweRelief** as needed, using up to 6 daily. **Caution:** *Do not use DLPA if you have PKU. Do not use tyrosine if you take MAO inhibitor or tricyclic antidepressants, or if you have a history of a melanoma.*

Irritable Bowel Syndrome – 1 **Colon Balance** capsule, three times daily.

Skin problems – **Lysine** 1,000 to 3,000 mg daily along with Alpha Lipoic/Green tea cream.

Memory problems – **Huperzine A**, 1 (50 mcg) capsule in the morning and in the evening. **Caution:** *Do not use Huperzine if pulmonary problems or Congestive Heart Failure exist, or if you are pregnant or lactating.*

PeriMenopause women – 1 to 2 PhytoBalance capsules, twice daily between meals. **Caution:** *Do not use if pregnant or lactating.*

Chronic Pain

Chronic pain is America's most common, expensive, disabling, and overprescribed disorder. Research demonstrates that patients who suffer for long periods become very depressed. The longer you suffer, the greater the intensity of pain. Pain sends an estimated 120 million Americans to doctors, pain clinics, and chiropractors every year. Pain cripples our lives and drives millions to addictive prescription drugs and alcohol.

Every year, the American public spends 6 billion dollars for analgesics (painkillers) and therapies of every description, but they still experience pain. Pain is one of the most serious problems not only in the U.S., but in the world. Back pain afflicts 85 million, arthritis 56 million, migraines 30 million; and 900,000 live with the hell on earth of cancer pain.

There are no magic bullets, no miracle drugs, no overnight cures. If anyone tells you they have a cure for pain, run, don't walk away. If a physician tells you surgery is the answer, get a second opinion and then make sure they review all the potential postsurgical problems. If you are offered an array of medication, consider the long-term effects, because drugs treat only the symptoms. Your goal is to treat the source—your brain—the master controller that sends signals to every corner of the body!

Remember, whatever the brain tells the body to do, it does! Pain research at Johns Hopkins University indicates a great deal of chronic pain and depression reflects the patient's inability to produce enough of certain brain chemicals. This research points to new methods of treating pain and depression, without using harmful drugs.

Studies at other major universities have shown the brain does produce many hormone-like chemicals that have a close functional resemblance to morphine. These morphine-like chemicals are called endorphins (endogenous morphine) because they are produced by the body (endogenous), and are similar to morphine.

Endorphins regulate pain and control the transmission of pain signals. Endorphins are inhibitory neurotransmitters in the brain and nervous system. They slow down the transmission of pain information from the limbic system to the cortex. Endorphins and other neurotransmitters help link together the one-hundred-plus billion neurons of the human brain into an incredibly complex network. From this complex network come our natural painkillers, endorphins. Endorphins have been shown to be more powerful than morphine. Are they the answer to pain control? Yes and no.

Endorphins are not drugs, but a simple nutritional amino acid, phenylalanine. The pain studies involved DL-Phenylalanine, or DLPA. DLPA is not a drug. It does not actually block pain, itself. DLPA works by protecting your own naturally produced endorphins, effectively extending their life spans in the nervous system. By extending their life spans, pain relief results. DLPA is a natural healer, and helps the body heal itself. Depression loves pain, pain loves depression; but DLPA has the ability to elevate the brain chemistry so that you do not feel depressed and in more pain. DLPA can do this because it is an inhibitory neurotransmitter.

DLPA is now being used clinically throughout the U.S. in major pain clinics, for pain and depression. Millions of people suffering from pain do so because of stress. Stress energizes pain, pain fuels stress. We see patients every day taking a combination of pain medications and antidepressants for stress-induced pain. *Harrison's Principles of Internal Medicine* states 50 to 80% of all pain is stress induced. This means there is no pathology; the pain is there, but there is no disease.

Those who suffer from stress-induced pain are depressed and negative because they are low in 34 of the 36 neurotransmitters made from amino acids. Most amino acids, themselves, are pain-relievers, especially 5-HTP—a safe, natural way to boost serotonin levels. Serotonin is absolutely essential for smooth brain function. If you live with chronic pain, you are deficient in serotonin, and, therefore, are more sensitive to pain messages from the brain.

Suggested Nutritional Support

PoweRelief – 2 caps, two to three times per day. **Caution:** *Do not use if you have PKU, have had a melanoma, are pregnant or lactating, or if you use MAO inhibitors or tricyclic antidepressants.*

Mag MAXX Cream – Apply lightly as needed to painful

area. Mag MAXX contains proprietary blend of fatty acids, magnesium chloride, and boswella that reduce inflammation and pain.

Rodex Forte (time released) – 1 capsule before breakfast. Rodex Forte contain contains B6 (150 mg), B12 (200 mcg), and folic acid (800 mcg).

DHEA – 25 to 50 mg capsules first thing in the morning if over 40. **Caution:** *Do not use if you have had cancer.*

Mag Link – 1 to 2 tablets, twice to three times daily OR *Mag Chlor 90* – 15 to 25 drops, twice to four times daily, divided in small amount of water or juice. If no diarrhea or loose stools occur, try increasing to a total of six per day. *Take to bowel tolerance, then decrease by 1 tablet or 1 dosage if you are taking the liquid.*

Boswella Plus – 1 or 2 capsule(s), mid-morning and mid-afternoon.

DLPA 750 – Take 5 minutes after meals, 3 times per day. Keep in mind DLPA takes from 2 days to 3 weeks to take effect. If your doctor has prescribed medication, you do not have to stop taking it. DLPA can greatly enhance the effectiveness of aspirins and analgesics. **Caution:** *Do not use if you have PKU, have had a melanoma, are pregnant or lactating, or if you use MAO inhibitors or tricyclic antidepressants.*

Mood Sync – 2 capsules in the morning, and 2 in the evening. **Caution:** *Do not use if you are taking an SSRI, SNRI, tricyclic, or MAOI antidepressant, or have had a melanoma.*

Taurine 1000 – 1 capsule, three times per day.

Brain Link – 3 scoops in the morning.

GABA 375 or 750 – 1 capsule, two to three times per day.

ProDHA – 2 softgels, twice daily OR **Pure Fish Oil Capsules** – 1 softgel, twice daily. EFAs help reduce inflammation, a large part of pain by reducing the production of prostaglandins. **Caution:** *Do not use if you take anticoagulants (blood thinners), are allergic to iodine, or if you will have surgery within a week.*

SerraEnzyme 80,000 I.U. – Take 1 to 3 capsules, twice to four times a day or use

Curcumin x 4000 – Take 1 to 3 capsules daily for acute inflammation. **Caution:** *Do not use if allergic to soy, have gallstones, or blocked bile duct. Consult your doctor if taking anticoagulants (blood thinners).*

Glucosamine & Chondroitin – 500 mg capsule Glucosamine along with 400 mg Chondroitin, three times daily. Use glucosamine and chondroitin especially if your pain is related to a joint, your neck, or your back.

Easy C (Esterified C)– 1000 mg, four times per day.

5-HTP – Start with 1 (50 mg capsule or tablet) 30 minutes before bedtime; increase to 2, if needed. **Caution:** *If you are taking an SSRI, SNRI, tricyclic, or MAOI antidepressant, do not use 5-HTP OR use*

Melatonin – 1 (3 mg) capsule an hour before bed, for sleep.

Relaxation CD – Try to use a relaxation CD at least 30 minutes a day. If your muscles are relaxed, your muscles will not increase your pain with spasms.

Magnets – Use north pole accuband or north pole magnets applied to the area of pain to reduce inflammation and pain. The magnets can be used repeatedly without fear of addiction. If the magnets stop working, stop using them for a few day, then reapply and they will again work.

Depression

Depression is an intensely isolating experience that can lead to losing a positive self-image and self-worth. You feel lost and alone, and no matter how you try, you cannot seem to pull yourself up from the darkness. There is hope for the twenty million Americans suffering from chronic depression, the dark and lonely emotion.

Depression is very treatable without toxic antidepressant drugs. Antidepressants cause you to give up control and let the drugs block your feelings. Drugs cause you to live a passive existence. There is no such thing as a tranquilizer deficiency! The causes

Major Symptoms of Depression
- Passive negativity
- Oversleeping combined with chronic fatigue
- Constant indigestion
- Dry mouth
- Compulsive eating, especially carbohydrates
- Appetite loss or changes in eating patterns
- Constipation or diarrhea
- Inability to make decisions
- Loss of confidence or self esteem
- Frequent or unexplainable crying

of depression include genetic, biological, personality, environmental, and nutrient deficiencies. Stress related events may be the major cause of cell depression and events that occurred in early life can prime the limbic system for later depression.

Depression can coexist with other disorders both physical and psychological. Each disorder can feed off the other such as chronic pain, fibromyalgia, or headaches.

If you have a chemical imbalance causing your depression, you have a deficiency of norepinephrine or serotonin. These two neurotransmitters are the major neurotransmitters that control mood in the brain. Drugs work by manipulating these neurotransmitters usually by increasing the amounts of norepinephrine or serotonin.

Tyrosine, because of its role in assisting the body to cope physiologically with stress and building the body's natural store of adrenaline, deserves to be called the stress amino acid. Stress exhaustion needs tyrosine which is converted to dopamine, norepinephrine, and epinephrine. The use of tyrosine along with SBNC (Super Balanced Neurotransmitter Complex) in depression increases levels of serotonin and neurotransmitters. These help restore a sense of well-being.

Tyrosine was first used in psychiatry for medication-resistant depression. Dr. A. J. Gelenberg (1980), of the Department of Psychiatry at Harvard Medical School, used tyrosine to treat patients that presented with depression. These patients noted significant improvement with tyrosine.

5-HTP, or 5-Hydroxytryptophan boosts the serotonin levels in the brain and creates neurotransmitters that produce an inhibitory effect on the nervous system. 5-HTP is converted into serotonin in the brain. Serotonin soothes, calms, and gives you a warm feeling of contentment. If you have a deficiency of serotonin, symptoms of depression, obsessive-compulsive disorder, anxiety, pain, and migraines will be demonstrated. Recent studies show that 5-HTP is as effective as Prozac without the side effects when the two were compared. Both Mood Sync and Teen Link contain 5-HTP. Mood Sync is an inhibitory neurotransmitter support formula that boosts serotonin and dopamine levels in the brain to give you a balance mood. Mood Sync contains tyrosine, GABA, glutamine, 5-HTP, taurine, Vitamins C and B6.

L–T® or L-Theanine is a new amino acid that derives from green tea. It readily crosses the blood-brain-barrier. In 1999 a study published in the *Journal of Food Science and Technology* confirms theanine has a significant effect on neurotransmitter release of dopamine and serotonin, plus it increases alpha waves in the brain. The brain produces alpha waves in a deep state of meditation. This release decreases depression symptoms. L–T® produces a tranquilizing effect in the brain without drowsiness or a dull feeling.

In the *Archives of General Psychiatry,* research suggests that omega-3 fatty acids are the missing link in depression. Low levels of omega-3 fatty acids are seen in patients with major depression. Research suggests depressed individuals receive marked benefits with omega-3 supplementation without negative side effects.

In three randomized double blind controlled studies published in 2002 and 2004 showed positive outcomes in depressed patients on medications. The patients that received omega-3 fatty acid supplementation showed 50% improvement in their depressive score and 6 out of 10 patients improved compared to 1 in 10 in the control group. In addition to omega-3, patients took a minute amount of Vitamin E tocopherol.

People with allergies or high histamine levels will have chronic low-grade depression. Additionally for allergy sufferers, add 500 to 1,000 mg of methionine daily, divided doses, and BCAAs (Branched Chain Amino Acids), 500 to 1,000 mg, daily. These amino acids will help you feel better.

For information regarding SAMe, see methionine section.

Suggested Nutritional Support

Tyrosine 850 – For chronic depression, use 850 mg, twice daily. **Caution:** *Do not use If you are taking an SSRI, SNRI, tricyclic, or MAOI antidepressant or have a history of melanoma.*

B6 – 100 to 150 mg daily, preferably in timed-release form, such as Rodex Forte. Rodex Forte contains B6 (150 mg), B12 (200 mcg), and folic acid (800 mcg).

Mood Sync – 1 or 2 capsules, twice to three times daily. **Caution:** *Do not use Mood Sync if you are taking an SSRI, SNRI, tricyclic, or MAOI antidepressant, or have had a melanoma.*

Mag Link – 4 to 6 tablets per day, divided OR

Mag Chlor 90 – 15–25 drops in juice, 2 to 3 times daily. *If diarrhea or loose stools occur, take tablets or drops by spacing further apart or decrease dosage by 1.* Mag Link and Mag Chlor provides magnesium chloride, the same form of magnesium present in the body, so it is readily absorbed and tolerated.

GABA 750 – Use ½ capsule to 1 capsule three times daily, divided and dissolved in water. GABA levels of those with depression are usually low. This information surfaced in a study done by F. Petty, M.D., of the Department of Psychiatry, Veterans Medical Center in Dallas.

ProDHA – 2 to 4 softgels, twice daily OR **Pure Fish Oil Capsules** – 1 to 2 softgels, twice daily (EFAs). **Caution:** *Do not use if you take anticoagulants (blood thinners), are allergic to iodine, or if you will have surgery within a week.*

Neuro Links – 15 drops, 3 times daily, or as needed.

5-HTP – 2 at bedtime. **Caution:** *If you are taking an SSRI, SNRI, tricyclic, or MAOI antidepressant, do not use 5-HTP.*

L–T – 2 capsules, twice to three times daily.

Methionine – 1,500 mg, three times daily with 2 SBNC in the morning. For information regarding SAMe, see methionine section.

Probiotics (Acidophilus) – Give some daily to boost good bacteria in the gut. Recent research shows a connection between the gut, the head, and behavior.

SPECIAL NOTE about Depression

If the combination of Mood Sync and Tyrosine is not enough and you still experience depression, or if you have taken SSRIs for over a year, you might consider pure 5-HTP. Some people with low serotonin levels need the increased 5-HTP to obtain depression relief. If this is the case, use 50 mg of 5-HTP, two to three times daily along with 100 mg of 5-HTP at bedtime. Be sure to take B6 as the body requires it to activate your amino acids. Take some GABA or L–T along with the 5-HTP. *If you are currently taking a SSRI, or SNRI antidepressant, DO NOT take 5-HTP. If you experience drowsiness with the pure 5-HTP, go to the Mood Sync.* Always add EFAs to help lift your mood.

Children

For children under 100 pounds, use 500 mg **tyrosine,** once daily with 50 mg B6. If over 100 pounds, use 500 mg tyrosine, twice daily with 50 mg B6. **Caution:** *If you are taking an SSRI, SNRI, tricyclic, or MAOI antidepressant, or if you have a history of melanoma, do not use HTP10 or Teen Link.*

HTP10 – 1 capsule, twice daily, if under 100 pounds. If over 100 pounds, use 2 HTP10, twice daily, **Caution:** *If you are currently taking a SSRI, or SNRI antidepressant, DO NOT take 5-HTP or HTP10.*

Or Use **Teen Link** – 1 capsule, twice daily. **Caution:** *If you are taking an SSRI, SNRI, tricyclic, or MAOI antidepressant, or if you have a history of melanoma, do not use HTP10 or Teen Link.*

Teenagers

Teen Link – 1 or 2 capsules, twice daily. Always start with 1 capsule twice daily, and see if that lifts the depression. Only if depression is not eased, increase to 2, twice to three times daily. **Caution:** *If you are taking an SSRI, SNRI, tricyclic, or MAOI antidepressant, do not use Teen Link.*

Bipolar Disorder (Manic Depression)

Bipolar is an affective disorder with emotional swings between two extremes, mania and depression. Mania is characterized by excessive excitement or overly excited and extremely sad, hopeless, depression. Anxiety, depression, and elation are the three affects most commonly seen clinically, but usually the extremes of elation or depression are what are treated. Occasionally, a mixed mood occurs with symptoms of both mania and depression. Wide changes in energy, activity, sleep,

> ## Mania Symptoms
>
> - Mean age of onset is 30 occurring in both sexes equally
> - Feeling "high", excessively happy, or outgoing mood
> - Extreme irritable mood, agitation, feeling jumpy or wired.
> - Abrupt change in behavior
> - Easily distracted
> - Talks extremely fast and jumps from one idea to another
> - Insomnia
> - Restless, whirling mind
> - Impulsivity, high risk behaviors
> - Family history of bipolar and unipolar illness and possibly alcoholism.
> - Depressive
> - Extreme sadness, worrying or feeling empty
> - Loss of interest in once enjoyable activities including sex
> - Tired all the time
> - Hypersomnia
> - Restless or irritable
> - Thoughts of death, suicide or attempting suicide
> - Changes in eating, sleeping, and other habits
> - Difficulty with memory and concentration, remembering or making decisions

and behavior occur along with changes in mood in an individual that exhibits bipolar disorder. About 1% of the population suffers from bipolar disorder and usually begins in the teens, 20s, and 30s.

Suggested Nutritional Support

Since bipolar disorder is a balancing act between mania and

depression, it is best to use a 2 sided nutritional approach.

Maintenance nutrients for Balance

Pure Fish Oil Capsules – 1 to 2 softgels, twice daily (EFAs). **Caution:** *Do not use if you take anticoagulants (blood thinners), are allergic to iodine, or if you will have surgery within a week.*

5-HTP – 2 at bedtime. **Caution:** *If you are taking an SSRI, SNRI, tricyclic, or MAOI antidepressant, do not use 5-HTP.*

L–T – 2 capsules, twice to three times daily to help stabilize mood.

Methionine – 1,500 mg, three times daily with 2 SBNC in the morning. For information regarding SAMe, see methionine section.

Lithium Orotate – 1 (130 mg) capsule (providing 4.8 mg elemental lithium), twice daily. **Caution:** *Do not use if you renal or cardiovascular disease, use diuretics, ace inhibitors or are pregnant or lactating.*

B6 – 100 to 150 mg daily, preferably in timed-release form, such as Rodex Forte. Rodex Forte contains B6 (150 mg), B12 (200 mcg), and folic acid (800 mcg).

Mag Link – 4 to 6 tablets per day, divided OR

Mag Chlor 90 – 15–25 drops in juice, 2 to 3 times daily. *If diarrhea or loose stools occur, take tablets or drops by spacing further apart or decrease dosage by 1.* Mag Link and Mag Chlor provide magnesium chloride, the same form of magnesium present in the body, so it is readily absorbed and tolerated.

Neuro Links – 15 drops, 3 times daily, or as needed.

Probiotics (Acidophilus) – Give some daily to boost good bacteria in the gut. Recent research shows a connections between the gut, the head, and behavior.

Mania episode nutrients

GABA 750 – Use ½ capsule to 1 capsule three times daily, divided and dissolved in water. GABA levels of those with mania and depression are usually low as revealed in a study done by F. Petty, M.D., of the Department of Psychiatry, Veterans Medical Center in Dallas.

SBNC — 1 to 2 capsules in the morning and afternoon.

Depressive episode nutrients

Mood Sync – 1 or 2 capsules, twice to three times daily. **Caution:** *Do not use Mood Sync if you are taking an SSRI, SNRI, tricyclic, or MAOI antidepressant, or have had a melanoma.* OR

5-HTP – 1 capsule, three times a day and 2 at bedtime. If depression still exists, increase to a total of 6 per day. **Caution:** *Do not exceed 6 per day. If you are taking an SSRI, SNRI, tricyclic, or MAOI antidepressant, do not use 5-HTP.*

SBNC — 1 to 2 capsules in the morning and afternoon.

Diabetes

Approximately 10 million Americans have diabetes. Diabetes is a chronic disorder of carbohydrate, fat, and protein metabolism. Diabetes occurs when the pancreas does not secrete enough insulin, or if the cells of the body become insulin resistant. As a result, blood sugar is unable to get into the cells. Diabetes can lead to multiple serious medical complications.

There are two basic types of diabetes: Type 1 and Type II. Patients with Diabetes Mellitus, or Type I, are insulin-dependent. This most often occurs in children and adolescents. Type II usually begins after the age of 40. Type II diabetics are non-insulin dependent, and comprise 90% of all diabetics.

According to Julian Whitaker, M.D. in his book *Reversing Diabetes*, some of his patients with Type I diabetes report having very stressful events in their lives that occurred six months to a year before they developed diabetes. Stress can alter the immune system, causing it to weaken. This predisposes an individual to the disease state, and often the onset of diabetes.

Besides regulation of blood sugar, antioxidants are extremely important for anyone with blood sugar issues. Antioxidants fight free radicals that cause damage to tissues in the body, causing aging. Cardiovascular disease (CVD), heart, and kidney problems are major concerns for the diabetic or anyone with Syndrome X. The eyes are very vulnerable to free radical damage, so protect your eyes by taking antioxidants on a daily basis.

Minerals are extremely important for diabetics. Essential minerals include magnesium, vanadium, selenium, zinc and manganese. Minerals help the body repair the mitochondria, particularly the organelles that regulate the mitochondria. Manganese and selenium are important for helping the body to neutralize free radicals and to produce SOD (Superoxide Dismutase). Vanadium is an important trace mineral that helps blood glucose regulation. You may have to cut back on your oral medications. In one study patients were given 50 mg of Vanadium, twice daily. The patients were moderately obese diabetics and non-diabetics. Decreases in fasting blood glucose and significant improvement in insulin resistance was noted with Type 2 diabetics with no change in non diabetics. Vanadium improves hemoglobin A1C also.

All diabetes are deficient in magnesium. Magnesium is involved in over 300 enzyme reactions in the body, muscle relaxation, sleep, and more.

Other nutrients that help repair the mitochondria are the branched chain amino acids (BCAA). Valine, Isoleucine, and Leucine comprise the BCAAs. But the BCAAs make up 20% of all muscle proteins. Muscle loss is common among diabetics, but the BCAAs assist blood sugar metabolism as well as reducing muscle loss.

Suggested Nutritional Program

Always use capsule, powder, or liquid form for maximum absorption.

Anxiety Control 24 – 1 or 2 capsules, twice per day, or as needed to decrease stress and anxiety.

Chromium Picolinate – 600 mcg daily, divided to help regulate blood sugar and decrease insulin resistance.

Gymnema Sylvestre – 300 mg, three times daily, divided before meals. Gymnema Sylvestre is a herb that aids in controlling sugar uptake and cravings. Two studies showed favorable effects from GS by lowering postprandial glucose plus improved glucose tolerance. In one study GS promoted regeneration of some pancreatic beta cells (cells that produce insulin) and an increase in insulin levels. GS needs to be taken constantly for 6 to 12 months to lower blood glucose levels, especially in Type 1 diabetics. Use care if you add GS because it may lower your blood sugar.

Mag Link – 4 to 6 tablets per day, divided OR

Mag Chlor 90 – 15–25 drops in juice, 2 to 3 times daily. *If diarrhea or loose stools occur, take tablets or drops by spacing further apart or decrease dosage by 1.* Mag Link and Mag Chlor provide magnesium chloride, the same form of magnesium present in the body, so it is readily absorbed and tolerated.

Vanadium – 50 to 100 mg per day, divided. Use the lowest amount of vanadium that keeps your blood sugar under control. You may have to cut back on your oral medications. Do this under the supervision of your physician.

Carnitine – 2 (250 mg) capsules, twice per day. Carnitine is important in fat distribution in the body. It helps reduce cholesterol and triglyceride levels to normal in the body and may improve insulin sensitivity

Fish Oil – 2,000 to 4,000 mg daily (2 to 4 softgels). Fish oil supports good total cholesterol levels in the body. Fish oil decreases total cholesterol while improving HDL/LDL (high density lipids to low density lipids) ratios since it inhibits the body's synthesis of cholesterol. Additionally, fish oil reduces inflammation thereby lowering cardiovascular risk. Fish oil greater than 4 grams per day may increase bleeding. Fish oil is an alternative to aspirin that is commonly recommended by cardiologists to reduce risk of heart attack. **Caution:** *Do not use if you take anticoagulants (blood thinners), are allergic to iodine, or if you will have surgery within a week.*

Fiber – helps keep blood sugar in the normal range. Use 2 tablespoons of Fortified Flax in any food or beverage. Fortified Flax provides 4600 mg of Omega 3 (good oil) needed on a daily basis.

Rodex Forte – 1 timed-release capsule in the morning that contains B6 (150 mg), B12 (200 mcg), and folic acid (800 mcg).

Taurine – 500 to 1,000 mg capsule, twice daily aids the release of insulin.

Deluxe Scavengers (antioxidants) – 3 per day, divided. Deluxe Scavengers combines CoEnzyme Q10, beta-carotene, Vitamins C, and E, Lemon bioflavonoids, rutin, Selenium, Glutathione, NAC, riboflavin, and Vitamin B6 as P5'P.

Easy C (Esterified C) – 2,000 to 3,000 mg per day, divided. Vitamin C is vital for the repair of all body tissues and scavenger of free radicals in the body.

Vitamin E – 400 to 800 I.U. daily. Vitamin E is important for the circulation, heart, neurological functions, and scavenging free radicals.

Manganese – 15 mg daily. Manganese is important for pancreas repair.

Decaf Green Tea Extract – 2 (500 mg) capsules, twice daily for antioxidant and anti-inflammatory properties.

CoEnzyme Q10 – 80 to 120 mg (in capsules) per day. CoQ10 supports the immune system, helps provide increased oxygen to the heart and body, and acts as a protective factor for the heart.

Alpha-Lipoic Acid (ALA) – 300 mg, twice daily; ALA is an antioxidant and especially important for diabetic neuropathy.

Branched Chain Amino Acids (BCAA) – 500 mg capsule daily.

Eat as many fruits and vegetables as possible, using organics, if possible. Fiber helps stabilize blood sugar, and reduces the need for insulin. Complex carbohydrates are more slowly metabolized so blood sugar levels increase more slowly.

Amino Acids and the Elderly

Many factors contribute to how quickly we age. The combined effects of genetic inheritance, health habits, medical history, life-style, sociocultural background, and environment all play a part in our aging. Many of the elderly do not take the time to cook nutritional foods. Therefore, they deplete their immune system and illness prevails.

Senior citizens are more prone to fatigue, dizziness, and falls, as their muscles do not respond as quickly as they did when they were younger. Sudden movements or exertion can increase the probability of falls.

The heart muscle begins to wear out from the stress of everyday life. The muscle becomes less elastic with age from exposure to free radicals found in air, sun, and environment. Cardiac output is reduced due to thickening and hardening of the heart valves and chambers. The overall consequences reduce oxygen delivery to the cells. In addition, plaques of fat build up in our blood vessels and arteries.

Elasticity loss in the lungs reduce vital capacity. Damage from free radicals stiffens the exchange sacs called alveoli. As a result, the air exchange is compromised,

Ingestion % of Daily Value in People Over 60					
	M	F		M	F
Vitamin B6	66	72	Vitamin D	51	62.5
Vitamin B12	19	31	Calcium	20	35
Folic Acid	54	72	Zinc	40	67

Function, Cognition, and Behavior Influenced by Nutrients

Nutrient	Influence
Taurine	Seizures
Carnitine	Cognition, depression
Phenylalanine	Catecholamines, dopamine, depression
5-HTP (Tryptophan)	Sleep, serotonin, neurotransmitters
Thiamin (B1)	Carbohydrate sensitivity
Riboflavin (B2)	Neurotransmitter control, neuropathy
Niacin (B3)	Dementia
Pyridoxine (B6)	Neurotransmitter cofactor
Cobalamin (B12)	Dementia
Folic Acid	Dementia
Choline	Memory, acetylcholine synthesis
Inositol	Peripheral neuropathy
Pantothenic Acid	Fatigue
Vitamin E	Parkinson's disease
Iron	Neurophysiological problems
Magnesium	Sleep disturbances, nervous exhaustion
Zinc	Smell, taste
Copper	Neurotransmitter control, RBC formation

affecting the health of the body tissues.

As a person ages, their ability to digest proteins diminishes. The amount of stomach acid-and protein-digesting enzymes decreases. Up to 30% of people over 60 do not secrete any stomach acid. Since most people over 60 have a decreased ability to digest proteins, and proteins are broken down into amino acids, then supplementation with amino acids will provide a base to cover the essential amino acids needed by the body. Since enzymes decrease with age, a pancreatin supplement with each meal facilitates the digestion of foods.

The digestion and elimination process slows down as we age. Poor appetite is a common complaint, due to many factors. Salivary secretion decreases by 50 to 60%. Loss of teeth, or gum disease, makes chewing more difficult and painful. Constipation may result from decreased fluid intake, lack of fiber, little or no exercise, and decreased intestinal motility.

Probably one of the most apparent changes occurs in the skin. The skin loss of resiliency and wrinkling becomes very evident. The skin becomes drier, thinner, more fragile, and less elastic.

The bones begin to break down through bone demineralization, reduced exercise and activity, and loss of calcium from kidneys and intestines. The loss of height becomes apparent in many seniors. The mineral loss in bones makes the bones more fragile and brittle. Sometimes the bones break, causing a fall.

Nutritional status influences all parts of the nervous system. The neurotransmitters regulate the physiological processes, and the way the brain processes information relates to our nutritional status. In several studies done on individuals 65 and over, the results indicate cognitive tasks corresponded to the nutritional status of the individual.

Alterations in psychological and neurophysiological performances occur when a person is deprived of, or low in, the B vitamins. As an example, acetylcholine derives from the B complex vitamin, choline. Inadequate amounts of choline can affect the synthesis, release, and metabolism of acetylcholine, and alter nerve function. Serotonin, an inhibitory neurotransmitter derived from tryptophan, decreases with age. Conversely, the catecholamine family—epinephrine, norepinephrine, and the neurotransmitters derived from phenylalanine or tyrosine—decreases with aging. These changes can produce mood swings, depression, and sleep-pattern alterations.

The nutritional status based on a person's unique genetic needs, determines cognitive and behavioral functioning.

In the past decade researchers have realized the relationship between the activity and function of the nervous system to the availability and metabolic activity of various nutrient-derived substances, including amino acids, vitamins, minerals, essential fatty acids, and other conditionally essential nutrients such as carnitine, taurine, and glutamine.

Between 50 to 60% of the brain is fat. This fat is not stagnant. Replacement of this fat occurs at the rate of 2 to 8% per day for DHA and 3 to 5% for arachidonic acid (AA). In patients with Alzheimer's, other dementias, and cognitive impairment deficiencies of EFAs (DHA, EPA, total omega-3 fatty acids) lower the omega-3 to omega-6 ratio. The ratio of omega-3 to omega-6 needs to stay in balance. Most Americans consume more omega-6 fatty acids (AA) due to meat consumption. Consumption of more omega-6 promotes inflammation that may lead to more disease.

Dementias occur more frequently in seniors and the brain is not able to make the connections it did previously. Alzheimer's is the most commonly occurring. The second most common type of dementia is called vascular dementia. In the traditional medicine model, there is no standard treatment available. Dementia symptoms include depression or flat affect, delayed thinking and speech, insomnia or excessive somnolence.

Vascular dementia develops when impaired blood flow deprives parts of the brain cells food and oxygen. It may occur after a stroke, or a series of small strokes or infarcts that block small blood vessels. Sometimes these strokes occur and are not noticeable, but over time the combined effects become apparent. Impairment may occur gradually or quite suddenly with cognitive or language changes. Sometimes after general anesthesia in seniors,

> **Vascular Dementia Symptoms**
>
> Memory problems
> Flat mood
> Confusion
> Difficulty concentrating
> Difficulty speaking or finding the word to speak
> Reduced ability to carry out activities of daily living
> Difficulty solving problems
> Lack of interest in areas that were previously enjoyed
> More difficulty with reading and writing

vascular dementia develops. Regional anesthesia or a local is the safest and carry the least risk for adults, especially seniors. Sedation helps to allay anxiety and helps block the experience.

Arginine is an important amino acid for seniors. Arginine fights infections, wound healing, fatigue, vasodilates blood vessels increasing blood flow to the heart, and acts as a neurotransmitter in the brain that participates in learning and memory.

Suggested Nutritional Support (Over age 60)

For all seniors, always use powder, liquid or capsule form. Never take in tablet form, as tablets do not break down as readily, so absorption is impaired.

SBNC – 2 capsules, a.m. and p.m. ⎫
B Complex – 1 capsule, twice per day. ⎬ *USE ALL THREE TOGETHER*
T– L Vite – 1 capsule in the morning, ⎭

Or use **Brain Link Complex** – 2 scoop in the morning, and 2 scoops in afternoon in juice.

Deluxe Scavengers (antioxidants) – 1 capsule, three

times per day.

CoEnzyme Q10 – 50 mg to 100 mg, once per day.

Mag Link – 4 to 6 tablets per day, divided OR use

Mag Chlor 90 – 15–25 drops in juice, 2 to 3 times daily. *If diarrhea or loose stools occur, take tablets or drops by spacing further apart or decrease dosage by 1.* Mag Link and Mag Chlor provides magnesium chloride, the same form of magnesium present in the body, so it is readily absorbed and tolerated.

ProDHA – 2 softgels, twice daily OR **Pure Fish Oil Capsules** – 1 to 2 softgels, twice daily. **Caution:** *Do not use if you take anticoagulants (blood thinners), are allergic to iodine, or if you will have surgery within a week.*

Acetyl-L-Carnitine (ALC) – 1,000 to 2,000 mg daily. ALC stimulates acetylcholine an important neurotransmitter for memory and for connecting brain cells. ALC improves focus and concentration while lifting the mood slightly. ALC protects the brain against oxidation and deterioration by inhibiting cell death.

Sea Buckthorn – 1 capsule twice daily helps fight aging. Sea Buckthorn is one of the most powerful antioxidants available.

Arginine – 1,500 to 5,000 mg per day depending on need. See arginine section for dosage details and balance with lysine.

Cal, Mag, Zinc Complex with Vitamin D and Boron – 4 capsules at bedtime. The latest research shows that Vitamin D is vitally important in multiple processes in the body from bones, muscles, skin, cancer preventative, etc.

5-HTP – For sleep, 1 or 2 capsules an hour before bedtime, with a piece of fruit. Always start with 1 capsule, increase to 2, if needed. **Caution:** *If you are taking an SSRI, SNRI, tricyclic, or MAOI antidepressant, do not use 5-HTP* OR use

Melatonin – For sleep, 1 (3 mg) capsule, an hour before bed.

Liquid Serotonin – 10 to 20 drops, as needed, for agitation or insomnia.

Neuro Links – 15 to 20 drops under the tongue as needed

to help restore neurotransmitter levels.

DHEA – 1 (50 mg) capsule upon arising in the morning. **Caution:** *Do not use if you have a history of cancer.*

Pregnenolone – 1 (50 mg) capsule, upon arising in the morning.

Green Tea Extract (Decaf) – 2 capsules twice daily for antioxidant and anti-inflammatory properties.

Fortified Flax – For constipation, start with 1 teaspoon twice per day, dissolved in fruit juice. Increase up to 1 tablespoon, if needed OR use

Phosphatidylserine (PS 100+) – 100 mg, three times per day, if cognitive functions are deteriorating.

Huperzine – 50 mcg capsule, twice daily to increase memory and concentration. **Caution:** *Do not use Huperzine if pulmonary problems, asthma, or congestive heart failure exist, or if you are pregnant or lactating.*

Galantamine (GalantaMind) – for Alzheimer's like symptoms, add 4 mg daily for a week. After 1 week, add a second 4 mg capsule. If desired, after another week, add a third or total of 12 mg per day.

Probiotics (Acidophilus) – Take some daily to boost good bacteria in the gut. Recent research shows a connections between the gut, the head, and behavior.

Grief

Grief is an equal opportunity affliction and a universal human experience. No one is immune to it, and everyone will be affected at some time in their life. The symptoms of grief are many, and the grieving process is a slow and painful process. Grief is an extremely individual experience. The symptoms of grief behavior are extensive. These behaviors can be described under four general categories.

A) Feelings B) Physical symptoms
C) Cognitive D) Behaviors

In grief, you experience a wide range of mental symptoms and feelings including depression, denial, anger, anxiety, fear, uncertainty, etc., but expressing these emotions is sometimes difficult. In the beginning grief and depression overwhelm you. You feel out of control. Over time, you work through the various stages of grief. The intensity of grief is interrelated to the degree of attachment to the person and your relationship with them, the level of understanding and support you receive from others, your personality and the nature of the bereavement. Eventually, you move forward with your life, but you fall back. Appetite disturbance presents a major problem and can cause long-term illness, if not addressed properly and corrected. In grief, your neurotransmitter level becomes very low from the prolonged stress and anxiety. Grief can cause fuzzy or irrational thinking, as well as avoidance behaviors. Many people refuse to let go or close the casket,

Physical Sensations Most Commonly Experienced from Grief

- Hollowness in the stomach
- Tightness in the chest
- Tightness in the throat
- Oversensitivity to noise, bright lights, and certain smells (such as hospitals)
- Detached from reality
- Breathlessness or shortness of breath
- Muscle weakness
- Fatigue
- Dry mouth
- Waking up several times nightly
- Appetite changes
- Chronic pain
- Headaches

and go on with their life. You are trying to keep that person alive. Staying in the past with a loved one causes anxiety and phobias as well as physical illnesses.

Ultimately, you are able to create a new life arising from the old. Remember, at all stages of grief, your brain and body need extra support. Your neurotransmitter levels exhaust, and you must replenish in order to move forward.

Note: Find a therapist you can talk to and whom you feel comfortable sharing your feelings. See him/her at least weekly through your acute stage, then on a monthly basis for the first year, and then as needed. Do not repress your feelings. Allow them to flow. If you took care of a loved one during a long illness, you can take on their symptoms which can include fear, depression, as well as their physical pain. Close the casket. Say good-bye, and let them go. *Otherwise, your healing cannot begin.*

Suggested Nutritional Support

Adults

Mood Sync – 1 or 2 capsules, twice to three times per day, in acute stage; and then 1 to 2, twice per day, as maintenance.

Grieving Process

For those who cared for a sick relative, grief and depression hit harder and longer. A study sponsored by the National Institute of Mental Health found 30% of caregivers suffer from clinical depression or anxiety while their loved one is alive. Four years later, 25% still suffered symptoms. Of those 25% still suffering, 50% experienced sleeplessness, 61% depression, 41% back pain, and 24% stomach problems. Only 10% of non-caregiving *relatives were depressed four years after death.*

Caution: *Do not use If you are taking an SSRI, SNRI, tricyclic, or MAOI antidepressant, or have had a melanoma.*
OR Use **Tyrosine** – 500 mg, 2 to 3 times daily, spread throughout the day. **Caution:** *Do not use If you are taking an SSRI, SNRI, tricyclic, or MAOI antidepressant, or have had a melanoma.*
B6 – 50 mg in the morning.
Brain Link Complex – 1 serving in the morning.
OR Use **T–L Vite** – 1 in the morning with breakfast.
5-HTP – 50 mg capsule, 1 hour prior to bedtime. **Caution:** *If you are taking an SSRI, SNRI, tricyclic, or MAOI antidepressant, do not use 5-HTP.*
Liquid Serotonin – Use 10 to 15 drops as needed throughout the day.
Mag Link – 2 tablets, twice daily OR use
Mag Chlor 90 – 15–25 drops in juice, 2 to 3 times daily. *If diarrhea or loose stools occur, take tablets or drops by spacing further apart or decrease dosage by 1.*
Anxiety Control – For acute episodes of anxiety, 1 or 2 capsules twice to three times daily, divided, as needed.
Taurine 1000 – 1 capsule, twice daily.

Children

Brain Link Complex – use 1/2 scoop in juice, in the morning.
Tyrosine – 200 to 500 mg depending on weight, daily. Under 50 pounds, use 200 mg. **Caution:** *Do not use If you are taking an SSRI, SNRI, tricyclic, or MAOI antidepressant, or have had a melanoma.*
Liquid Serotonin – Use 6 to 10 drops as needed throughout the day.
Anxiety Control – 1 capsule, mid-morning, afternoon, and 30 minutes before bedtime.
Taurine 500 – 1 capsule, twice daily.

Teenagers

Teen Link – Use 1 or 2 capsules, twice daily. **Caution:**

Do not use If you are taking an SSRI, SNRI, tricyclic, or MAOI antidepressant, or have had a melanoma.
Brain Link Complex – 1 serving in the morning, and 1 in the evening.
Taurine 1000 – 1 capsule, twice daily.

Other Factors
- **Avoid sugar and do not use alcohol** for depression.
- **Avoid prolonged periods in dark rooms** or rooms with drapes closed except when sleeping.
- **Probiotics (Acidophilus)** – Take some daily to boost good bacteria in the gut. Recent research shows a connections between the gut, the head, and behavior.

Grief from Pet Loss

Your pets become part of your family, and when their lives come to an end, you can experience deep feelings of grief and loss. There is no set time for your grief, or for how long it will last. Don't be ashamed to express your feelings of loss. Your pet intertwined with the daily rhythms of your life, especially when you first came home, at meals, and at bedtime. You experience the same deep, lost, and lonely feelings you do with a human loss. When a beloved pet dies, part of your lifestyle is lost. All that your pet symbolized is lost—comfort, love, companionship, security, and joy.

Pets accept you unconditionally. They allow you to express any emotion. They don't judge, or criticize; they just love and accept. When the loss occurs, many of us feel confused by the deep level of grief, because your pet was part of your family and lived each hour of each day to give you love. Don't suppress your feelings. Allow them to flow so you can put closure on your loss, and allow the healing process to begin. Use the nutritional support program outlined, as long as needed.

Grief support groups include:

- **Pet Partners (formerly Delta Society)** (425) 679-5500 Monday through Friday, 8:30 a.m. to 4:30 p.m., Pacific time. Website: www.petpartners.org They specialize in counseling those who have lost a pet and need assistance with their grief. Check with the Delta Society's web site at http://www.deltasociety.org for the latest info about support and pet grief groups.
- **ASPCA (American Society for the Prevention of Cruelty to Animals)** National Pet Loss Hot line at 1-877-474-3310. The hot line is available 24/7 and is answered by a psychologist. If she has another call or is traveling, you may have to leave a message.
- Support Service – **Companion Animal Association of Arizona** Inc. P.O. Box 5006, Scottsdale, AZ 85261-5006. **Pet Grief Support Help line:** (602) 995-5885. Association Number: (602) 258-3306. Operated entirely by trained volunteers the service provides understanding, compassion, and support to persons throughout the U.S. and Canada who are anticipating or coping with the loss of a beloved companion animal. The Service offers a 24-hour-a-day telephone help line, regularly scheduled support group meetings, information, literature, and reading lists on pet loss, and referral to appropriate resources. Although there is no charge for the Service, long-distance calls to the Help line will be returned collect. Companion Animal Association website is www.caaainc.org.
- **Michigan State University Pet Loss Hot line** – Phone: (517) 432-2696. Tuesday and Thursday 6:30 p.m.-9:30 p.m. EST.
- **Cornell University Pet Loss Hot line** – Tuesday, Wednesday, and Thursday 6 p.m.-9:00 EST Phone: (607) 253-3932. Website: www.cornell.ed/org/Petloss. Click on *Other Hot lines* for pet loss referrals in FL, IL,

IA, MA, MI, VA, WA.
- **Tufts University** – Phone: (508) 839-7966. During the academic year: Monday-Thursday 6:00 p.m.-9 p.m. EST. During the summer: hours vary, call for information. If someone is not available, leave a message and your call will be returned during the next normal hot line shift. Email for non-urgent matters: Tuftspetloss@gmail.com Email is only checked sporadically. If you want to speak to someone regarding pet loss, call the above number.

Headaches

Headache is the number one complaint of the American public. Consumers spend approximately 6 billion dollars per year on pain medications and over-the-counter formulas for relief. It is estimated that yearly approximately 90% of men and 95% of women suffer from headaches painful enough to send them to doctors' offices. The source of the headaches is not located in the brain itself, as there are no sensory nerves in the brain. Pain produced inside the skull is rare and usually due to tumors or other disorders; the pain is a secondary symptom. Most headache pain originates outside the skull in the nerves leading to the muscles and blood vessels around the face, scalp, and neck.

The most common types of headaches include migraine, tension or muscle contraction, and cluster. Often, a person can experience a combination of headaches. But headaches may also be caused by other underlying problems, such as sinus or allergy.

Food or stress can trigger migraines. Migraines are often called the avoidance headache. Migraine headaches produce a throbbing pain on one side of the head, but the pain can spread to the entire head. Often nausea and sometimes vomiting occur. Visual symptoms are common. Facial tingling or numbness may occur. Other symptoms include extreme sensitivity to noise and lights. Usually the attacks last from 4 to 72 hours without treatment, and commonly interfere with normal activity to some extent. Migraine sufferers may look pale and feel cold. Sometimes the victim gets a forewarning of an attack with malaise, fatigue, and mood changes. It is not uncommon for the sufferer to feel exhausted and mentally foggy for hours after an attack.

Headache triggers include:

- Stress, anxiety, anger, or depression
- Menstruation, oral contraceptives, or hormone-replacement drugs
- Foods such as dairy, MSG, eggs, anything pickled, alcohol (beer or red wine), coffee, teas, chocolate, wheat, cheese, or tomatoes are the most common. But any food can be a culprit. Explore food allergies as a contributing cause. There are lab tests for differentiating foods, or you can do a food-elimination diet.
- Environmental substances such as perfumes, paint, new carpet, glues, fumes, etc., or strong smells
- Missed or delayed meals
- Flickering fluorescent lights, sunlight
- Time-zone changes
- Holidays and travel
- Loud noises
- Bone structure misalignment and muscle spasms with trigger points
- Alteration of sleep-wake cycle, such as sleep deprivation or excesses
- Certain drugs
- Wine, especially red wine and other alcoholic beverages
- Low magnesium levels

Tension or muscle-contraction headaches are probably the most common form of headaches. Tension headaches account for 75% of all headaches, and are usually a response to stress, fatigue, or environmental factors; they can even start after a stressful event. The pain in the head results from muscle contractions of the head, neck, back, or facial muscles. Pain is often felt in the forehead, extending up from the base of the skull. The muscles of the upper back or neck contract, causing the pain to refer to the head. This is frequently described as a tight feeling, like a band or vise around the head. The neck and shoulders often feel sore, and the person can develop trigger points in the muscles. Trigger points are sore, tender points that form scar tissue within the muscle. The trigger point causes the muscle to go into contraction from stress, anxiety, overuse, poor posture, or staying in the same position for an extended period of time. The headaches can become chronic and occur daily. Headaches can last only a few minutes, but usually last several days. Nausea is uncommon with muscle-contraction headaches, and usually do not limit activities as do migraines. But muscle-contraction headaches can make you feel that you are going crazy from the pain. The chronic muscle-contraction headache can bring on depression, anxiety, and sleep problems. Massage with deep-tissue work sometimes benefits. But if the muscle does not let go, it may be necessary to have trigger point injections to break up a headache. Consider osteopathic or chiropractic manipulation for chronic headaches.

    The most important supplement for 90% of headaches is magnesium. At the Pain & Stress Center the best results with headaches and pain were seen with magnesium chloride (Mag Link or Mag Chlor). Mag chloride addresses the needs of your body at cellular level. Absorption and tolerance was best with magnesium chloride orally and intravenously.

    Cluster headaches cause very severe one-sided head pain. Usually the pain centers in the eye. Other symptoms include excessive tearing, drooping eyelid, stuffy or runny nose, all on the side of the pain. Restlessness is a common symptom. The pain can be so severe that the sufferer paces or bangs their head against the wall to contend with the headache. Cluster headache attacks usually last 30 to 90 minutes, but they can last hours. The sufferer generally has recurrent attacks over a month to three months, with the headaches occurring during an active phase once or twice daily, or every other day. Then the headaches do not recur for several months to years. There is no known cause for cluster headaches.

About 90% of headaches are due to the aforementioned. Other most common causes of headaches include the following:

- Sinus headache. Due to increased pressure in the sinus cavities; often a sinus infection. Sinus headaches last until the sinuses drain. A sinus infection should be treated with antibiotics.
- Temporomandibular Joint Dysfunction (TMJ). Usually occurs in the temple, ear, or cheek regions of the head. Caused by clenching of the jaws, or grinding of the teeth. (Usually at night or from abnormalities of the jaw joint itself. Stress intensifies TMJ pain).
- Glaucoma. Increased intraocular (eye) pressure. Acute glaucoma may cause a throbbing pain around or behind the eye, or in the forehead. Eye redness and vision of halos or rings around lights may occur with glaucoma.
- Hypertension. Increased blood pressure; can contribute to a headache.
- Strokes, aneurysms and brain hemorrhages. A severe headache of sudden onset associated with stupor, or other neurological symptoms, demands prompt medical evaluation.
- Head trauma can cause pain, and can reflect serious damage ranging from fractured skull to internal bleeding.
- Occipital neuralgia headache. Occurs mainly in senior

citizens. Symptoms include jabbing pain in the back of the head and neck, tenderness in neck and shoulder area.
- Other miscellaneous causes of headache include eyestrain, allergies, dental problems, dehydration, systemic infections, caffeine withdrawal, meningitis, brain swelling, and intense physical exertion.

If you have persistent pain that does not respond to rest and treatment, consult a physician. If you experience a headache accompanied by severe pain, drowsiness, confusion, mood swings, visual disturbances, weakness or paralysis, consult a physician immediately.

Suggested Nutritional Support for Headaches

PoweRelief Capsules – 1 or 2 caps every 4 to 6 hours, as needed, for relief. PoweRelief combines DLPA, Boswella, GABA, Ashwagandha, and B6. **Caution:** *Do not use PoweRelief if you have PKU, are pregnant, lactating, have a history of melanoma, or if you take MAO inhibitor or tricyclic antidepressants.*

DLPA 750– 1 or 2 capsules, twice per day. **Caution:** *Do not use DLPA if you have PKU. Do not use DLPA if you take MAO inhibitor or tricyclic antidepressants, or if you have a history of a melanoma.*

Boswella (300 mg) – 1 or 2, twice per day. Boswella is a herb from India, used for inflammation or swelling.

Anxiety Control – 2 capsules, twice to three times per day.

Mag Link – 4 to 6 tablets per day, divided OR use

Mag Chlor 90 – 15–25 drops in juice, 2 to 3 times daily. *If diarrhea or loose stools occur, take tablets or drops by spacing further apart or decrease dosage by 1.* Magnesium can also be given I.V. for acute headache and migraines. Mag I.V. usually produces quick relief.

Mood Sync – 1 or 2 capsules, two to three times daily. **Caution:** *Do not use If you are taking an SSRI, SNRI, tricyclic, or MAOI antidepressant, or have had a melanoma*

L–T – 2 capsules, twice daily. At bedtime, open 2 capsules and dissolve in small amount of water. Then add 20 drops of Mag Chlor for a nighttime sleep cocktail in 6 ounces of fruit juice.

Riboflavin – 400 mg daily for migraine prevention. Be patient as it may take up to 2 months to notice a difference according to Dr. Stephen Silberstein, director of the Jefferson Headache Center at Thomas Jefferson University in Philadelphia.

Alka-Seltzer Gold – 2 tablets dissolved in a glass of water at onset of a migraine headache. Often, this brings immediate relief for migraine headaches triggered by allergic reactions to food or chemical substances. The Alka-Seltzer Gold helps to neutralize the allergic mechanism, and prevents the migraine from becoming full blown.

Accuband Magnets – Use on trigger points on the neck and upper back to relieve pain. Accubands are tiny, powerful magnets about the size of the top of a pencil eraser that are applied with a small adhesive patch. These tiny magnets begin to ease pain immediately. **Caution:** *Do not use if pregnant, have pacemaker, or implanted medical device.*

B Complex – 1 capsule in the morning.

Mag MAXX™ Cream – Apply to neck and back once or twice per day, or as needed.

NAC – For sinus congestion/headache, 1 (600 mg) capsule, twice daily.

Other Suggestions for Sinus Headaches

- Elevate head above waist.
- Apply ice pack to base of neck and on upper shoulders for 20 minutes at a time, then off for 30 minutes. Repeat as needed.
- Avoid heating pad for muscle-contraction or migraine headaches.
- For sinus headache, apply hot, moist towels, or apply a specially designed moist heating pad to the sinuses to facilitate sinus drainage.

- Massage to neck and shoulders can help relieve headache.
- Irrigate your sinuses with a bulb syringe or a nettie pot with a mixture of saline with 2,000 mg of MSM.
- Consider medical evaluation for possible sinusitis or sinus infection and trigger point injections, if headache persists.

Heart Disease

Heart disease or coronary heart disease (CHD) is the number one killer of Americans, and causes half the deaths in the U.S. today. An estimated 57 million Americans are afflicted with some type of heart disease. Heart disease claims over 720,000 people each year.

Your sex, family history, and age pose risk factors beyond your control. But the other risk factors you can control. The most dangerous are high cholesterol, hypertension, and smoking. Each risk factor increases the risk of having a heart attack 2 to 3 fold, and all the risk factors compound each other dramatically.

Studies have shown that high cholesterol levels are directly proportional to your risk of heart attack. Diet is the next highest component that determines your cholesterol level. Dean Ornish, M.D., has proven cholesterol and your risk of heart disease can be dramatically changed with dietary and lifestyle changes, and love. Be aware, if you do not eat enough fat or cholesterol, the body increases the production of cholesterol in the liver. The body interprets the reduction of fats or cholesterol in the diet to a time of famine or starvation. This causes insulin to activate HMG Co-A reductase, an enzyme in the liver, to manufacture more cholesterol than is required by the body from sugars and carbohydrates.

Cholesterol lowering drugs work by inhibiting the

Risk Factors for Heart Disease
- Male gender, or postmenopausal women
- Genetics, history of heart disease in family
- Age
- High blood cholesterol
- Hypertension or high blood pressure
- Diabetes
- Smoking
- Excess weight
- Lack of exercise

HMG Co-A. Many cholesterol-lowering medications also lower the CoEnzyme Q10 level and can cause liver damage. This can put you at higher risk for having a heart attack. CoQ10 is an enzyme necessary for cell oxygenation, and is essential for health of all tissues and organs in the body. As we age, the CoQ10 level drops dramatically. CoQ10 helps protect against heart attacks, relieves angina, boosts the immune system, lowers blood pressure, is an antioxidant, and helps periodontal disease.

Hypertension or high blood pressure afflicts 35 million, or 1 in 6 Americans. If hypertension is present, the likelihood of CAD is 3 to 5 times higher than if the person has normal blood pressure. It is important that you have your blood pressure checked by a health care professional, at least twice yearly. Recently, studies demonstrate that arginine is an important factor with heart disease and hypertension.

Research suggests that inflammation plays a large factor in cardiovascular disease, atherosclerosis, and hypertension than previously thought. Elevation of C-Reactive Protein (CRP) is a major risk factor for heart disease, stroke, peripheral vascular disease, and cardiovascular death. The H-S CRP (High Sensitivity C Reactive Protein) is the strongest single predictor of the risk of cardiovascular events.

If you have had a heart attack, add D-Ribose to your regiment. Heart scans have shown that D-Ribose revitalizes areas of the heart that were damaged from the restriction of blood flow to your heart muscle when you had your heart attack. D-Ribose decreases the recovery period from a heart attack to over exercising, and even, reduces the amount of heart damage, if given right away following a heart attack. In addition, D-Ribose helps congestive heart (heart failure) patients utilizing 3,000 mg of D-Ribose, twice daily.

Smoking is the third controllable risk factor. Quit! A complete nutritional program is outlined in our *Break Your Prescribed Addiction* book. Your risk of a heart attack one year after you quit smoking is just 10% greater than the nonsmoker; after 5 years of abstinence, your risk factor becomes the same.

Suggested Nutritional Support

Carnitine – 1,000 to 3,000 mg per day, divided, for high cholesterol and triglycerides. Carnitine also increases the HDL (good) cholesterol. Immediately after a heart attack, supplement with 2 grams of carnitine to facilitate expansion of the heart muscle again. Continue carnitine at the 2 gram level. This reduces heart muscle damage while lessening angina and arrhythmias (abnormal heart rhythms).

Taurine – 1,000 mg, three times daily, and may be increased up to 6 grams per day, if needed. Taurine is the most abundant amino acid in heart tissues. Taurine increases left ventricle function without changing the blood pressure, and helps balance the calcium and potassium in the heart. But Taurine also lowers blood pressure (vasodilates blood vessels), improves insulin sensitivity, and reduces homocysteine levels.

Mag Link – 4 to 6 tablets per day, divided throughout the day OR use

Mag Chlor 90 – 15–25 drops in juice, 2 to 3 times daily.

If loose stools occur, decrease the dose by 1, or try spreading out the interval between doses. If you have CAD or hypertension, you are deficient in magnesium. Magnesium is nature's muscle relaxant, and is vital to a healthy heart. Mag Link is a magnesium chloride, the same form of magnesium found in the body's cells; absorption and tolerance are best with this form of magnesium.

Chromium Picolinate – 200 mcg, per day. Chromium helps lower total cholesterol and triglycerides, while raising HDL cholesterol.

Vitamin E (preferably mixed tocopherols)– 400 to 800 I.U., per day. Vitamin E is an antioxidant. Recent studies demonstrated a lower risk of fatal heart attack, if Vitamin E is taken daily.

DHEA – 25 to 100 mg per day, upon arising in the morning, on an empty stomach. (Have your physician check your DHEA sulfate level to obtain a starting point, and then have it checked 2 to 3 months after starting DHEA). In patients with CAD, the blood levels of DHEA have been very low; i.e., DHEA sulfate level of 4 (normal is 250—900). If you are over 50, start with 25 mg if you are a female, and 50 mg if you are male. Recheck your DHEA levels and adjust accordingly and consider adding Pregnenolone (PG) 50 to 100 mg and let your body determine how much DHEA your body needs. PG is the precursor for DHEA. Your body will produce the DHEA it needs. **Caution:** *Do not use DHEA if you have had cancer, especially uterine or prostate.*

CoEnzyme Q10 – 100 mg, per day, for CHD or hypertension; this may be increased to 225 mg per day. For congestive heart disease, increase CoEnzyme Q10 to 300 to 500 mg, per day, plus magnesium and B6. **Caution:** *If you are take large doses of CoQ10, you need to remain on that dosage or decrease very slowly.*

Deluxe Scavengers – 3 per day divided. Deluxe Scavengers are a combination formula comprising CoEnzyme Q10, beta-carotene, Vitamin C, Lemon bioflavonoids, rutin, Vitamin E, Selenium, Glutathione, NAC, riboflavin, and Vitamin B6 as P5'P.

Easy C (Esterified C) – 2,000 to 5,000 mg per day, divided.

Garlic – 1,500 to 3,000 mg, divided. Garlic is an alternative to aspirin therapy. Ajoene, a component of garlic, is at least as potent as aspirin.

Folic acid – 400 to 800 I.U., daily. Folic acid is necessary for the proper metabolism of homocysteine. Excess homocysteine causes arterial plaque buildup.

Anxiety Control – 1 or 2 capsules, twice or three times daily, as needed for anxiety or stress.

L–T – 2 capsules, twice to three times daily for anxiety and to lower blood pressure. L–T is excellent to take with Mag Chlor as a bedtime cocktail to sleep more restfully.

Rodex Forte – 1 capsule in the morning, for hypertension and congestive heart failure. Rodex Forte contains B6 (150 mg), B12 (200 mcg), and folic acid (800 mcg).

Decaf Green Tea Extract (DGTE) – 2 capsules, twice daily. DGTE is a super antioxidant, inflammation fighter, while fortifying your immune system.

SerraEnzyme 80,000 I.U. – 1 to 2 capsules, twice to four times daily to reduce inflammation.

Hawthorn – 1 to 1.5 grams freeze-dried berries, three times daily. Hawthorn improves the circulation of blood to the heart by dilating blood vessels and relieving arterial spasms.

ProDHA – 2 softgels, twice daily OR

Pure Fish Oil Capsules – 1 softgel, twice daily. **Caution:** *Do not use if you take anticoagulants (blood thinners), are allergic to iodine, or if you will have surgery within a week.* DHA and EPA, omega-3 fatty acids, decreases blood-platelet stickiness, lowers triglycerides, lowers blood pressure, and reduces inflammation.

Arginine – 5,000 mg, twice daily per Dr. Mark Houston, a Professor of Cardiology at Vanderbilt University. Arginine assists arterial blood vessels to release nitric oxide and it improves the blood vessels' abilities to dilate. Sherry Rogers, M.D. calls Arginine, the nitroglycerin of the body.

Take Arginine with at least 3,000 mg of lysine + 1,000 mg of **Easy C** (Esterified C), twice daily, if you have problems with herpes outbreaks.

Alpha Lipoic Acid – 300 mg, twice daily.

Sea Buckthorn – 1 capsule twice daily helps fight aging. Sea Buckthorn is a super antioxidant along with essential fatty acids.

D-Ribose – 1 scoop (about 2 tsp.) twice daily with morning and evening meal. D-Ribose is essential to the body's energy production that is a crucial building block for cell synthesis of ATP (adenosine triphosphate) or cell energy. This helps in tissue recovery and strength. D-Ribose supports healthy muscle function, supports exercise endurance while assisting in alleviation of muscle soreness and stiffness. D-Ribose facilitates energy reserves required to preserve cardiovascular health and wellness.

Other Factors

Exercise.

Paleolithic diet that consists of low sodium, high potassium, high fiber, low fat, lean animal protein, low refined carbohydrates, and low cholesterol intake such as fruits, vegetables, berries, nuts, fish, fowl, wild game, and other nutrient dense foods. Avoid the "whites," white flour, sugar, white breads, sugar, rice, etc. Use bread sparingly.

Celery – 4 stalks per day or the equivalent in celery juice, oil, or celery seed extract reduces high blood pressure. Luteolin (tetra-hydroxyflavone) in celery has the ability to heal or repair the peroxisomes. Peroxisomes are cells that often damaged by environmental plastics.

Reduce and avoid sugar. Sugar drives your triglycerides upward and plays a factor with your cholesterol.

Hepatitis C

Hepatitis C is a disease of the liver caused by the hepatitis C virus (HCV), and is the most common chronic blood-borne infection in the U.S. About 230,000 new infections occur each year according to the C.D.C. HCV usually results from direct percutaneous exposures to blood. HCV usually causes chronic inflammation of the liver.

The chances of persons with HCV infection developing long term infection, chronic liver disease, cirrhosis, liver cancer, or dying as a result of hepatitis C are:

- 55-85% might develop long-term infection.
- 70% might develop chronic liver disease.
- 5-20% might develop cirrhosis over a period of 20 to 30 years.
- 20% might die from long-term infection (liver cancer or cirrhosis).

Chronic liver disease is the tenth leading cause of death in U.S. adults accounting for about 25,000 deaths a year with 40% or 8,000 to 10,000 of these deaths related to HCV.

Dr. Burton Berkson, a physician and researcher from Las Cruces, New Mexico, has successfully treated Hepatitis C with supplementation. Dr. Berkson used Alpha Lipoic Acid or Thioctic Acid intravenously to regenerate the liver. Selenium acts as birth control for Hepatitis C while Silymarin protects against further liver damage. Silymarin is an antioxidant, blocks toxins at cellular level, has anti-fibrotic, anti-inflammatory, and immunomodulating activities.

The following are Dr. Berkson's suggestions for Hepatitis C in his triple antioxidant approach.

Suggested Nutritional Support

Alpha Lipoic Acid (pharmaceutical grade) – 300 mg, twice daily.

Selenium – 200 mcg, twice daily.

Silymarin (Milk Thistle) – 6 (300 mg) capsules per day.

B Complex – 1 capsule, twice daily. B Complex is needed to replace depleted thiamine, niacin, riboflavin, and biotin.

Other Helpful Supplements

Decaf Green Tea Extract – 2 capsules, twice daily.

NAC (N-Acetyl Cysteine) – 1 capsule, three times daily. NAC is a precursor to glutathione, a powerful detoxifying agent.

Easy C (Esterified C) – 2 capsules (500 mg), twice to three time daily.

Vitamin E – 400 to 800 I. U. daily.

CoEnzyme Q10 – 30 to 50 mg daily.

T-L Vite (good multi-vitamin and mineral) – 1 capsule with main meal.

ProDHA – 2 softgels, twice daily OR **Pure Fish Oil Capsules** – 1 softgel, twice daily. **Caution:** *Do not use if you take anticoagulants (blood thinners), are allergic to iodine, or if you will have surgery within a week.* DHA and EPA, omega-3 fatty acids, decreases blood-platelet stickiness, lowers triglycerides, lowers blood pressure, and reduces inflammation.

Anxiety Control – 1 or 2 capsules, twice or three times daily, as needed for anxiety or stress OR

L–T – 2 capsules twice to three times daily for anxiety and antistress. Since L–T derives from green tea, it also contains antioxidant properties. L–T is excellent to take with Mag Chlor as a bedtime cocktail to sleep more restfully.

Mood Sync – 1 or 2 capsules, two to three times daily for low mood or depression. **Caution:** *If you are taking an SSRI, SNRI, tricyclic, or MAOI antidepressant, do not use Mood Sync.*

Other Factors

High fiber diet with an abundance of preferably organic fruits and vegetables, low fat meats, and whole grains. Avoid salty or high iron foods.

Exercise and stress reduction.

Moderate sunlight for Vitamin D.

Stop smoking and harmful drugs.

Avoid alcohol ingestion and volatile hydrocarbon

solvents (e.g., gasoline).
Avoid excessive acetaminophen (Tylenol).
Avoid food additives.
Avoid foods that contain mycotoxins (aflatoxin, cyclosporine, etc.) Mycotoxin literally means "fungus poisons." Mycotoxins are toxins produced from fungus growth such as on peanuts, grains, cheese, and even black pepper.
Avoid general anesthesia.

Herpes

Herpes has become a major social disease. Herpes attacks are characterized by clusters of clear, fluid-filled vesicles on the genitalia or face, accompanied by severe pain and itching. Once a person becomes infected with the herpes virus, rarely will the virus become extinct. The virus rests dormant in the body after the initial infection. When it reactivates as a result of stress, such as emotional upset, sunburn, etc., the virus produces an outbreak. Stress causes reemergence of the virus, and changes the balance of the amino acids, arginine and lysine.

Keeping the balance of lysine to arginine at the right levels prevents replication of the herpes virus, and keeps it in check. Lysine is relatively easy to get in the diet, and most people consume ten times the minimum. However, vegetarians tend to have low lysine levels. A key to keeping herpes under control is to watch the ratio lysine-to-arginine foods. You must find the proper balance for you by trial and error. Avoid arginine-rich foods: chocolate, carob, coconut, oats, peanuts, soybeans, wheat germ, gelatin. Increase lysine foods: beef, chicken, lamb, milk, cheese, beans and brewer's yeast. In addition, take lysine supplementation in amounts of 500 to 1,500 mg per day.

Suggested Nutritional Support

Lysine – 500 to 1,500 mg per day as maintenance. During acute outbreaks, increase the lysine up to 6,000 mg, per day, and add another 1,000 mg of Vitamin C as Easy C (Esterified C). The following schedule for lysine works well for acute outbreak when you feel an outbreak coming on or after acute stress.

Day 1   1,500 mg twice a day
Day 2–7   5,000 to 6,000 mg spread throughout the day.
Day 8   2,000 mg in the morning and 2,000 in the evening
Day 9   1,500 mg twice a day
Day 10   maintain with 1,500 daily, divided.

Easy C (Esterified C) with Bioflavonoids – 500 mg, three to four times per day.

B Complex – 1 capsule, daily.

Lysine Cream – Apply to sores at onset, and repeat three to four times per day.

PoweRelief – 1 or 2 capsules, twice per day, as needed for pain. PoweRelief contains DLPA, boswella, ashwagandha, GABA, magnesium, and B6. **Caution:** *Do not use PoweRelief with DLPA if you have PKU, are pregnant or lactating, if you take MAO inhibitor or tricyclic antidepressants, or if you have a history of malignant melanoma.*

Mag MAXX cream – helps relieve discomfort of herpes. Apply topically as needed to affected area. Be sure to wash hands after applying to keep from spreading.

Emu Oil – apply topically for relief from herpes discomfort. Emu is an excellent anti-inflammatory while providing relief that quickly penetrates the skin. Be sure to wash hands after applying to keep from spreading.

Vitamin E – 400 I.U. capsule, daily.

Zinc – 60 mg per day for acute outbreak until healed; then 15 mg per day for maintenance. Zinc is important to skin.

Anxiety Control – 1 or 2 capsules, twice daily for acute stress or anxiety. During an acute outbreak, increase to three times per day OR

L–T – 2 capsules twice to three times daily for anxiety and antistress.

Mood Sync – 1 or 2 capsules, two to three times daily for low mood or depression. **Caution:** *If you are taking an SSRI, SNRI, tricyclic, or MAOI antidepressant, do not use Mood Sync.*

Mag Link – 4 to 6 tablets per day, divided OR use

Mag Chlor 90 – 15–25 drops in juice, 2 to 3 times daily. *If diarrhea or loose stools occur, take tablets or drops by spacing further apart or decrease dosage by 1.*

Other Factors

Ice Cube – If you feel tingling on an area around your mouth, apply an ice cube to the area for 5 minutes, then off for 5 to 10 minutes; repeat several times daily. This interrupts the virus' replication cycle, and may prevent a blister formation.

Immune Health

The immune system simply keeps us well. The immune system protects our body against all invaders— viruses, bacteria, parasites, cancer cells, etc., and recognizes them as foreign or not within the body. Immune system must be able to differentiate between self and foreign bodies defending against these foreign invaders. The body defends itself by calling into action components of the immune system, tonsils, spleen, thymus, adenoids, lymphocytes (lymph cells), white blood cells, and bone marrow, appendix, lymph nodes, and lymphatic network.

If the body overreacts, an error occurs that may lead to a sensitivity or allergy to a particular substance. For example, exposure to pollen from grasses, weeds, or trees may lead to sensitivity and allergy to that pollen. The body overreacts to the foreign substance calling into action the immune system, but fails to recognize the substance as an allergy. The body reacts by releasing histamine and calls into action, lymphocytes that cause an inflammatory reaction. If the reaction is severe, the individual may go into an anaphylactic reaction that can be life threatening. Since everyone is different, why someone reacts to particular pollens or develops cancer probably lies in the genes. Boost your immune system to help stay healthy.

Although some of the following are not amino acids, the nutrients and minerals are so important to health and they needed to be included in this book.

Vitamin D

Recently, many studies verify the need for Vitamin D in the body. Vitamin D is extremely important for staying healthy and the *most potent immunomodulator* according to Dr. Michael Holick. Vitamin D helps keep bones strong as well as your immune system. While the body can make Vitamin D if exposed to as little as 10 minutes of sun daily, many Americans do not or are not able to make the necessary amount of Vitamin D the body requires. About 40 to 60% of Americans do not have enough Vitamin D. Individuals with dark skin, living above latitude 35, elderly, ill, or use sunscreen need to supplement to obtain adequate levels of Vitamin D. Have your doctor run a 25-hydroxyvitamin D [25 (OH)D] to see if the level of Vitamin D is adequate. Normal 25-OH level (Vitamin D) is 60 to 80 ng/ml in a healthy, young individual. The medical community discourages sun exposure due to the risk of melanoma, but the risk is higher for the immune system, bones, cancers, and other diseases with low levels of Vitamin D. If you are over the age of 60, the amount of Vitamin D taken should be doubled the average adult to 4,000 I.U. daily. Average dosage for an adult is 2,000 I.U. daily. Over age 60, the body does not convert the Vitamin D to a usable form in the liver and kidneys as readily, so you require more to compensate.

Vitamins C and D might be called the wintertime infection fighters. These two vitamins fight the constant bombardment of germs and virus when our bodies are attacked. Of course, adding some green tea helps to fortify your body's defenses and ward off symptoms and infections. For more information about Vitamin D, read the *UV Advantage* by Michael Holick. Dr. Holick is a professor of medicine, physiology, and biophysics at Boston University and has studied Vitamin D for over 30 years.

Iodine

Another important mineral is iodine. According to the National Health and Nutrition Examination Survey between 1971 and 2000, the iodine levels in the U.S. declined by 50%. During this period of time, cancers of the breast, prostate, endometrium (uterus), ovaries increased along with increased thyroid illnesses (hypo), autoimmune rose. About 90% of the worldwide population

---

Drugs that Interfere with Vitamin D
- Anticonvulsants
- Anti-tuberculous drugs
- Bile salt sequestrants
- Digoxin
- Glucocorticoids (Steroids)
- Hydroxychloroquine (used for Lupus)
- Statins

is deficient in iodine and over one-third of the world's population lives in an iodine deficient region.

Iodine is found in every cell of the body or utilizes iodine. Iodine concentrates in the glandular system, especially the thyroid, breasts, salivary glands, parotid glands, pancreas, cerebrospinal fluid, brain, stomach, skin, and lacrimal (eye) glands. Iodine is an alkalinizing agent (elevates body pH), antibacterial, anticancer, antiparasitic, antiviral, and mucolytic (capable of reducing viscosity of mucus) agent. In 1918 researchers demonstrated that feeding rabbits iodine prevented cholesterol deposits in arteries that were fed cholesterol. More studies were done with iodine and comparable results were reported in medical literature.

Iodine seems to be a key factor for so many diseases yet the U.S. intake is very low. Sources of iodine include iodized salt, sea salt, seaweed, kelp, and ocean fish such as cod, sea bass, haddock, perch, etc. Iodine helps keep you healthy. Take some everyday. Recommended daily value is at least 150 mcg daily. But most people need 6 to 50 mg of iodine per day.

Recently, iodine has come to life resulting from the problems with the nuclear power plant in Japan after the earthquake and tsunami. Supplementing with iodine causes the body to uptake iodine rather than the

Iodine Deficiency is a Worldwide Problem Resulting in

- Mental impairment, mental retardation, reduced intellectual ability, ADD
- Goiter
- Infertility
- Increased risk of breast, endometrial (uterus), ovarian, prostate and other cancers

radioactive iodine released from the nuclear reactors, and helps protect against cancer and other immune disorders resulting from exposure to radioactive iodine.

Probiotics

You were not born with good bacteria in your intestines. At birth your immune system is weak and your gut is void of any good bacteria. Ingestion of mother's milk and other foods eaten later helped you obtain the good bacteria that you require for life. The bacteria multiply and attach themselves to your intestinal wall and thereby making your immune system strong. As you grow so does your bacteria flora. By adulthood, you have between 3 and 5 pounds of intestinal bacteria (flora). In the *Journal of Evolutionary Biology,* a 2009 study found that some of the healthy bacteria resided in your appendix. The appendix is often considered a non-essential organ, but research has shown that the appendix is actually a storage place for intestinal flora.

Most of the bacteria come from two genuses, either Lactobacillus or Bifidobacterium. These two bacteria help increase immunoglobin A (IgA) that strengthen your ability to fight off germs and viruses. These bacteria also decrease inflammatory chemicals, produce antimicrobial substances and improve the intestinal lining helping to prevent intestinal infection and food allergies.

You need normal flora to assist in the digestion of foods so it can be absorbed. If you do not have enough beneficial flora, your intestines become overrun with Candida albicans yeast, parasites, and other bad bacteria. A lack of good bacteria often results in yeast infections, urinary tract infections, fatigue, skin problems, IBS (Irritable Bowel Syndrome), chronic fatigue, indigestion, diarrhea, heartburn, and jock itch.

Antibiotics are the robbers of your intestinal flora. Antibiotics kill not only bad bacteria, but your good bacteria as well. It is vital that you replenish your supply of the good bacteria. Eat yogurt, kefir milk, or take a supplement that contains at least 10 to 40 billion CFUs per day to help restore your intestinal fortification and keep your immune system strong.

Suggested Nutritional Support

Easy C (Esterified C) with Bioflavonoids – 500 mg, three to four times per day. Exposure to pollen, increase to 1000 to 1500 mg, three to four times daily.

Beta Glucan (Immune Health Basics) – 75 to 500 mg, three to four times daily on an empty stomach at the first sign of illness. Only use intermittently to boost your immune system. *Do not stay on beta glucan continuously.*

SerraEnzyme 80,000 I.U. – 1 to 2 capsules every 4 to 6 hours helps to remove debris from the body that promotes inflammation and pain. Use intermittently for best results.

Green Tea Extract (Decaf) – 1 to 2 capsules twice daily for immune and antioxidant support. For more info on green tea, read our book, *Green Tea, Healing Miracle*.

Curcumin 500 to 1000 mg – 1 capsule every 6 to 8 hours to reduce inflammation. Curcumin is a potent antioxidant and phytonutrient. *Only use intermittently for best results.*

Olive Leaf Extract (d-Lenolate) – 1 to 2 capsules three times a day to help fight viruses and bacteria. *Only use d-Lenolate at intervals. Do not stay on continuously.*

Iodine 53 – 5 to 10 drops in water every day to boost your immune system and keep it healthy. *Do not use iodine if you are allergic to it.* OR use

Ioderol – 1 to 2 tablet every day to heighten your immune system. Start with 1 and gradually add second tablet. If heart rate accelerates, cut tab in half and start with one-half. *Do not use iodine if you are allergic to it.*

Daily D3 (as Cholecalciferol Vitamin D3) – 2, 000 to 5,000 I.U. daily.

Inflammation II (homeopathic) – 5 to 10 drops as needed to reduce inflammation and pain.
Anxiety Control or Mood Sync for stress support. Stress decreases your immunity. Support your brain and body with the needed neurotransmitters to keep healthy. Use 2 capsules, twice to three times daily of either Anxiety Control or Mood Sync. Use Mood Sync for down or volatile mood. **Caution:** *If you are taking an SSRI, SNRI, tricyclic, or MAOI antidepressant, do not use Mood Sync.*
Mag Link – 4 to 6 tablets per day, divided OR use **Mag Chlor 90** – 15–25 drops in juice, 2 to 3 times daily. Magnesium levels drop with stresses of any sort. *If diarrhea or loose stools occur, take tablets or drops by spacing further apart or decrease dosage by 1.*
Probiotics (Acidophilus) – Take some daily to boost good bacteria in the gut. Recent research shows a connections between the gut, the head, and behavior

Irritable Bowel Syndrome (IBS)

An estimated 20% of the American population suffers from Irritable Bowel Syndrome (IBS), a common functional bowel disorder for which there is no reliable medical treatment. IBS is a disturbance of the intestines, resulting in diarrhea, abdominal pain, and/or constipation. Patients suffering from IBS have increased sensitivity, not only to painful distentions in the small bowel and colon, but to normal intestinal functions as well. Stress, anxiety, or any type of emotional conflict will provoke symptoms of IBS. IBS responds to psychological, physiological, or dietary influences on the brain and body.

In his book, *The Second Brain,* Michael Gershon, M.D., Columbia-Presbyterian Medical Center in Bronx, New York, established that the stomach has a brain that functions independently. This second brain is located in the gut, and contains neurons, neurotransmitters, and proteins. According to Dr. Gershon, this may be why patients suffer from ulcers, chronic abdominal pain, gastrointestinal disorders such as colitis, and from nervous-stomach butterflies caused by anxiety or panic.

The gut's brain, known as the enteric nervous system, resides in the tissues that line the digestive organs. Dr. Gershon reports the gut contains 100 million neurons, as well as nearly every major substance found in the brain. This enteric nervous system also comprises major neurotransmitters such as GABA, neuropeptides, and enkephalins. As a second brain, it operates independently of the central nervous system; however, it interacts very closely with the body's other brain because of its connection with the vagus nerve. The vagus nerve can receive anxiety-, fear-, and panic-related stimulation from the limbic system in the head brain. Intestinal malfunctions such as diarrhea can result from repressed anger, hostility, or traumatic episodes. When the mind suffers, the body cries, and the entire nervous system responds with all the symptoms of IBS. Most of the serotonin in the body is produced in the gut or intestines and 60% remains in the gut. Only 1% of serotonin is produced in the brain.

People with multiple food sensitivities often experience symptoms of IBS. The primary offenders include dairy, wheat, and eggs. Other irritants involve coffee, corn, tea, citrus, some grains, and raw fruit. Once a person knows their food sensitivities, they can find useful fiber sources. Given the large number of people with wheat sensitivity, they can find relief with daily doses of the pleasant-tasting fortified flax. Fortified flax is rich in omega-3s, magnesium, fiber, and potassium.

Suggested Nutritional Support
Colon Balance – 1 capsule, three times daily. Colon Balance, a Chinese herbal formula, is a proven herbal

support formula for IBS.

Mag Link – 4 to 6 tablets per day, divided OR use

Mag Chlor 90 – 15–25 drops in juice, 2 to 3 times daily. *If diarrhea or loose stools occur, take tablets or drops by spacing further apart or decrease dosage by 1.* Mag Link and Mag Chlor provides magnesium chloride, the same form of magnesium present in the body, so it is readily absorbed and tolerated.

Anxiety Control – 2 capsules, as needed for stress and anxiety OR use **L–T** – 2 capsules twice to three times daily for anxiety and antistress. If you have a problem with depression and anger, use Mood Sync; 1 capsule, four times daily. **Caution:** *If you are taking an SSRI, SNRI, tricyclic, or MAOI antidepressant, do not use Mood Sync.*

Fortified Flax – 1 heaping teaspoon in the morning and in the evening.

Digestive Enzymes (i.e. Super Pancreatin) – 1 or 2 capsules with each meal.

Alka-Seltzer Gold – Use 2 tablets, dissolved in water, as needed for food reactions, bloating, or upset stomach.

Mint Tea (such as peppermint or green tea) – after meals, to aid digestion.

GABA 375 – Mix 1 capsule with a small amount of water and drink if your stomach is upset from stress or anxiety. The GABA helps calm the receptors in your stomach.

Decaf Green Tea Extract – 1 (500 mg) capsule twice a day to boost your immune system.

Melatonin – ½ to 6 mg, 30 minutes prior to bedtime. Melatonin possesses anti-inflammatory properties to help reduce intestinal inflammation. **Caution:** *Do not use melatonin if you are pregnant or lactating or less than 30.*

Probiotics (Acidophilus) – Take some acidophilus daily to boost good bacteria in the gut. Recent research shows a connections between the gut, the head, and behavior.

Insomnia

Sleep disorders affect about 80 million people in the U.S. NIH reports 18 to 20% of the American public suffers from insomnia. Insomnia is the perception or complaint of poor-quality, or inadequate, sleep. There are several forms of insomnia—the ability to fall asleep when you first go to bed; or constantly waking up during the night and being unable to go back to sleep. Waking up in the early morning, unable to return to sleep, in most cases is due to anxiety. Insomnia can be the result of varied causes, including pain, anxiety, depression, grief, stress, fear, caffeine consumption, stimulant drug use, and certain psychoactive drugs.

Insomniacs spent over 600 million dollars for prescription sleep products in 1999, and this grows at a rate of 20% per year. The National Sleep Foundation found, through a Gallup Survey, that approximately 75% of all Americans have trouble sleeping. At some point during our lives, up to 50% of Americans have at least one bout of chronic insomnia, but only 20% go to a doctor for treatment.

Many women with PMS, or those approaching menopause, can experience interrupted sleep patterns due to

Causes of Short-Term and Intermittent Insomnia

- Stress
- Environmental noise
- Temperature extremes
- Change in sleep environment
- Sleep/wake schedule problems
- Shift work
- Jet lag
- Medication side effects

Causes of Ongoing Insomnia

- Advanced age (>60 years)
- Female gender
- History of depression
- Stress/anxiety
- Medical problems
- Use of certain medications
- Chronic pain
- Low magnesium levels

hormonal imbalances. Millions of people suffer from a condition known as restless leg syndrome, or leg cramps. This condition, caused by a deficiency of magnesium, does not allow the muscles to relax, so they twitch and jerk all night. Magnesium deficiency can cause insomnia. Sleep apnea is a major problem and should be addressed by a physician who specializes in sleep disorders. If you have a problem with insomnia, do not consume any caffeinated coffee or beverage after 2 P.M.

Suggested Nutritional Support

5-HTP– 1 (50 mg) capsule, 30 minutes prior to bed, to elevate your serotonin level. Increase to 2, if needed. **Caution:** *If you are taking an SSRI, SNRI, tricyclic, or MAOI antidepressant, do not use 5-HTP.*

Mag Link – 4 to 6 tablets per day, divided OR use

Mag Chlor 90 – 15–25 drops in juice, 2 to 3 times daily. *If diarrhea or loose stools occur, take tablets or drops by spacing further apart or decrease dosage by 1.* Mag Link and Mag Chlor provides magnesium chloride, the same form of magnesium present in the body, so it is readily absorbed and tolerated.

Sleep Link – 1 to 2 capsules, 30 minutes prior to bedtime Sleep Link is a special combination of neuro nutrients that act as precursors to neurotransmitters. This formula includes melatonin, 5-HTP, GABA, glutamine, L-T (L-Theanine), Ashwagandha, Passion Flower, and P5'P (B6). **Caution:** *If you are taking an SSRI, SNRI, tricyclic, or MAOI antidepressant, do not use Sleep Link. Instead use melatonin and/or Mellow Mind.*

Melatonin – ½ to 6 mg, 30 minutes prior to bedtime. Continue using melatonin even if it does not seem to be work at first. Your circadian rhythm must be reset so it may take a week or two for your body to adjust, and for the melatonin to work properly. **Caution:** *Do not use melatonin if you are pregnant or lactating, or unless you are over 30 years of age. If you experience weird dreams or nightmares, you are taking too large a dose.*

Anxiety Control – 2 capsules, approximately 30 minutes prior to bedtime. If you wake up after a few hours, take an additional AC.

Mood Sync – 1 or 2 capsules, two to three times daily. **Caution:** *If you are taking an SSRI, SNRI, tricyclic, or MAOI antidepressant, do not use Mood Sync.*

Mellow Mind – 1 or 2 capsules, 30 minutes prior to bedtime. Mellow Mind contains 500 mg of Ashwagandha plus Esterified C.

Seditol – 1 capsule about one hour prior to bedtime. Seditol contains patented Magnolia Officinalis and Ziziphus jujuba that are Chinese herbs effective for sleep.

PoweRelief – 2 capsules, 30 minutes prior to bed, if you suffer from pain. Apply **Mag MAXX** lightly as needed. **Caution:** *Do not use PoweRelief with DLPA if you have PKU, are pregnant or lactating, if you take MAO inhibitor or tricyclic antidepressants, or if you have a history of malignant melanoma.*

Neurexan (homeopathic) – 1 to 2, as needed for sleep or restlessness at bedtime.

Other Therapies

- Always use capsules. Capsules break down more rapidly in the body, so you get to sleep more quickly.

Capsules do not contain fillers or binders, so they are generally a purer product. The one exception is Mag Link; it cannot be encapsulated due to its chemical structure.
- Play a relaxation CD to help you relax, and to promote sleep.
- Use deep-breathing exercises for 10 to 15 minutes, to relax the body and mind.
- Play some gentle, relaxing music an hour before you go to bed to allow your body to come down from your stressful day and prepare your body for sleep. Take a warm bath to relax your body for sleep.
- Avoid caffeine for at least 6 hours prior to bedtime.

Leaky Gut Syndrome

Leaky gut syndrome (LGS) is simply increased intestinal permeability. Someone with LGS exhibits many symptoms and illnesses. The precipitating causes of LGS include: abnormal flora (yeast, bacteria, parasites, etc.), food allergies, chemicals or drugs that irritate the small intestines or gut, chronic stress syndrome, and enzyme deficiencies, either genetic or acquired. At least 70% of our immune system is based on the health of our gut.

The digestive tract is vitally important for total body health. The intestinal tract, or gut, must be healthy or the rest of the body suffers. The digestive tract is a 25- to-30 foot-long tube that starts at the mouth and ends at the anus. The gut's function includes the digestion, into microscopic particles, of the food we eat, and absorption and conversion of these particles into energy. The intestine is responsible for absorbing vitamins and minerals into the bloodstream, detoxifying major chemicals in the body, and synthesizing antibodies and immunoglobulins that act as the first line of defense against infections. The intestine performs a dual function. As it allows nutrients into the bloodstream, it prevents large molecules, bacteria, other microbes, and toxins from entering. But the small intestinal mucosa has only a single-cell thickness.

A healthy gut lining allows properly digested proteins, fats, and carbohydrates to pass into the intestinal villi, or small fingerlike folds in the intestinal wall, while keeping out bacteria, large undigested molecules, and toxins. The gut repairs and replaces itself every three to six days. Leaky gut syndrome allows substances to pass through the intestinal lining that normally do not. Alcohol, foods, medications, and stress compromise the intestinal lining. These substances irritate and inflame the intestinal wall, and they cause tiny tears. The small intestinal lining develops large, leaky spaces between the cells of the intestinal walls, infringing the intestinal barrier, and allowing in bacteria, viruses, toxins, and foods. When there is a disruption of the normal intestinal flora, bacteria and fungus (yeast) overgrowth occurs, and immune-system resistance decreases. Normal flora disruption and increased intestinal permeability occur after surgery, nutritional tube-feedings, trauma from burns, severe blood loss, and other physical trauma.

The liver is the main organ that converts toxins or harmful substances into by-products that are excreted. Toxins can overload the liver. An overloaded liver does not detoxify, and allows extra toxins to enter the bloodstream.

Causes of Leaky Gut Syndrome

- Aging
- Antibiotics
- AIDS
- Candida
- Chemotherapy
- Chronic stress
- Chronic infections
- Environmental contamination
- Enzyme deficiencies
- Food allergies
- Gastrointestinal (GI) diseases
- Immune-system overload
- Overindulgence of alcohol
- Parasites
- Steroid medications
- Trauma

Symptoms Associated with LGS

- Abdominal pain
- Aggressive behavior
- Anxiety
- Asthma
- Bed-wetting
- Bladder infections (reoccurring)
- Bloating
- Candida
- Chronic joint pains
- Confusion
- Constipation
- Diarrhea
- Exercise intolerance
- Fatigue
- Fever of unknown reason
- Gas, upper and lower
- Indigestion
- Immunity poor
- Learning disorders
- Memory poor
- Mood swings
- Nervousness
- Muscle pains
- PMS
- Recurring infections
- Shortness of breath
- Skin rashes
- Fuzzy or spacey thinking
- Vaginal infections
- Yeast infections

A person with chemical and food sensitivities can develop autoimmune antibodies and more food and chemical sensitivities. You might assume the body is able to absorb more amino acids, vitamins, minerals, and nutrients, but, instead, your body absorbs less of these vital nutrients.

Antibiotics and nonsteroidal anti-inflammatory medications (NSAIDs) such as aspirin, Motrin (ibuprofen), and Aleve, cause LGS. Antibiotics do not discriminate; they kill both good and bad bacteria in the body and gut. Since antibiotics change the balance of the intestine, fungi (yeast), viruses, parasites, and resistant bacteria colonize the gut. These microbes contribute to inflammation, irritation, and leaky gut syndrome.

Steroids are used for allergies, asthma, autoimmune diseases, and inflammation. Long-term use of steroid medications, such as prednisone and nasal sprays for allergies, depress the immune system and encourage yeast infections in the gut.

Chronic stress also contributes to LGS by inhibiting the body's ability to heal or respond rapidly. Stress causes our bodies to secrete less DHEA, an adrenal hormone that possesses anti-aging and anti-stress properties.

Food sensitivities/allergies promote inflammation in the body, including the gut. LGS develops and allows food particles to enter the bloodstream. As foreign substances to the body, these food particles trigger an immune response. Ingestion of foods to which you are sensitive causes increased intestinal permeability. The insulted gut allows more food particles to pass into the circulation, and, as a result, you develop more food

Common Conditions Associated with Leaky Gut Syndrome

- Acne
- Aging
- AIDS
- Alcoholism
- Allergies /Asthma
- Ankylosing spondylitis
- Arthritis
- Autism
- Burns
- Candida infections (intestinal dysbiosis)
- Celiac disease
- Chemical sensitivities
- Chemotherapy
- Chronic fatigue
- Crohn's disease
- Cystic fibrosis
- Eczema
- Environmental Illness (EI)
- Fibromyalgia
- Food allergies/sensitivities
- Hyperactivity
- Inflammatory bowel disease
- Intestinal infections
- Irritable bowel syndrome
- Liver dysfunction
- Lupus
- Malabsorption
- Malnutrition
- NSAIDs ingestion
- Pancreatic insufficiency
- Nutritional deficiencies
- Poor diet
- Psoriasis
- Reiter's Syndrome
- Rheumatoid arthritis
- Trauma
- Ulcerative colitis

sensitivities as antibody responses.

If you have leaky gut syndrome, how do you get well? You must heal your gut; and you must be patient with yourself, as it will take time for your body to recover.

1) Remove the cause.
2) Restore good GI function by eating well, using a food-rotation diet if you have multiple allergies. If you know specifically the foods causing the problem, leave them out of your diet for at least four to six months, to allow the intestines to heal. Chew your food thoroughly and increase the fiber in your diet.
3) Eat a caveman diet. Eat fresh fruits and vegetables, nuts, seeds, and low-sugar foods.
4) Don't expect miracles from your body in one or two days. Be patient and persist, to help your body recover so you feel better and have a better quality of life.
5) Restore and help balance your gut bacteria with yogurt or kefir daily. Studies are showing that there is a connection between the gut, and the head, and plays a role in mental disorders.

Suggested Nutritional Support

Digestive Enzymes – Take 1 or 2 digestive enzymes, in capsule form, such as 2 **Super Pancreatin 650** capsules or Super Enzymes with each meal. The digestive enzymes help your body thoroughly digest ingested foods and to break down the foods into smaller particles, so they are less antigenic. *Always make sure your digestive enzyme is in capsule form;* tablets sometimes pass through your body without being absorbed.

Acidophilus – Take 1 or 2 acidophilus bifidus capsules, four times daily or eat yogurt or kefir milk. Reintroduce some good intestinal flora into the gut or intestine. If you are not allergic to milk, you can also take a teaspoon of "live-cultured" yogurt, twice daily. Other sources of acidophilus are non-milk yogurt and kefir milk.

Super Glutamine – Take 1000 mg of Super Glutamine (pure pharmaceutical grade powder), three to four times daily, to help repair the small and large intestines. The GI tract, especially the small intestine, is the greatest user of glutamine in the body. Glutamine is vital for our health.

Deluxe Scavengers – Take 3 capsules daily, divided. Deluxe Scavengers contain a mixture of the antioxidants in one capsule. This combination formula comprises CoEnzyme Q10, beta-carotene, Vitamin C, lemon bioflavonoids, rutin, Vitamin E, selenium, glutathione, NAC, riboflavin, Vitamin B6 as P5'P.

T-L Vite – 1 capsule with the main meal of the day.

Anxiety Control – 1 or 2 capsules, three to four times daily, for stress and anxiety OR

L–T – 2 capsules twice to three times daily for anxiety and stress.

Mood Sync – 1 or 2 capsules, three times daily for stress with depression. **Caution:** *If you are taking an SSRI, SNRI, tricyclic, or MAOI antidepressant, do not use Mood Sync.*

Easy C (Esterified C) – 2,000 to 4,000 mg, per day, divided.

Garlic – 1,500 to 3,000 mg, per day, divided. Garlic helps maintain a healthy intestine, promoting the proper bacteria in the gut.

Decaf Green Tea Extract – 1 or 2 capsules, twice daily to support your immune system.

Alka-Seltzer Gold – Use 1 tablet as needed to neutralize a food reaction. Any pharmacy can order it.

Probiotics (Acidophilus) – Get some daily to boost good bacteria in the gut.

Menopausal Stress/Anxiety

Menopause is simply the cessation of menses or periods. This occurs naturally in every female or suddenly with a hysterectomy. The menopausal path is often rocky with many ups and downs. Hormones become out of balance and the estrogen levels drops as much as 4 to 5 years before the last menstrual period. The average age of menopause is 51 years of age, but may occur anywhere from 30 to 60 years of age. Every woman can choose to get pregnant, but cannot escape menopause. PeriMenopause usually lasts 2 to 5 years, but you can experience symptoms as long as 10 to 15 years before menopause. You may feel like you are losing your mind and cannot remember not only where your keys were, but what you got up to get when you go across the room. And then there are the heavy periods, hot flashes, night sweats, insomnia, dryness, reduced sex drive, urinary/bladder urgency, and mood swings. These symptoms are not life threatening, but they are definitely challenging. Arguments exist in the medical community that many of these symptoms may be due to a lack of progesterone rather than a lack of estrogen. The drop in progesterone creates an estrogen dominance.

Many women experience anxiety and depression during PeriMenopause. You might notice more aches, pains and inflammation. Menopause brings new risks that can be life threatening. Foremost is a significant loss of bone mass that occurs in the first 5 to 7 years making you more vulnerable to osteoporosis. With the reduction

Effects of Estrogen Loss

- Hot flashes, night sweats.
- Dry skin and mucous membranes (includes vagina, nasal passages, mouth, and eyes)
- Loss of skin tone and elasticity
- Reduced sex drive and genital atrophy
- Memory loss
- Reduced sense of well-being
- Increased bone loss
- Hair thinning and loss
- Increased risk of heart disease, colon and breast cancers

Compounds of Plants with Estrogen-like Activity	
Phytoestrogen	Major Plant Source
Isoflavones	soy, beans, peas, spinach, fruits, cloves
Lignans	vegetables, fruits, nuts, cereals, spices
Flavones	green vegetables, beans, fruits and nuts
Chalcones	liquorice
Diterpenoids	coffee
Triterpenoids	licorice, hops
Coumarin	peas, spinach, cabbage and liquorice
Acyclic	hops

Source: Alan J. Husband, "Red Clover Isoflavone Supplements: Safety and Pharmacokinetics." *Journal of the British Menopause Society*, Supplement S1, 2001, p. 4

of estrogen, women are at risk for heart disease (coronary artery disease), and colon cancer.

Menopause causes major transitions for your body. You must be patient and allow your brain and body to adjust to all the changes. Using amino acids for stress, anxiety, and other menopausal changes lessens your fear, stress, anxiety, and uncertainty. Take control of your life.

Suggested Nutritional Support

T-L Vite – 1 capsule daily. T-L Vite is a multivitamin/mineral designed beneficial for postmenopausal women.

Mood Sync – 1 or 2 capsules, twice to three time daily for anxiety and depression. **Caution:** *If you are taking an SSRI, SNRI, tricyclic, or MAOI antidepressant, do not use Mood Sync.* Instead use Anxiety Control 2 capsules, three times daily, plus L–T,® 1 to 2 capsules, three times daily.

B Complex – 1 capsule, daily, in the morning with breakfast.

SBNC – 2 capsules, twice daily.

Sleep Link OR 5-HTP – 2 capsule (50 mg) an hour before bedtime, with juice. If needed, add 1 melatonin 3 mg capsules or a 500 mg Mellow Mind (Ashwagandha). **Caution:**

If you are taking an SSRI, SNRI, tricyclic, or MAOI antidepressant, do not use Sleep Link or 5-HTP. Instead use Anxiety Control, 2 capsules and a 3 mg Melatonin capsule, 30 minutes before bed.

ProDHA – 2 softgels, twice daily OR **Pure Fish Oil Capsules** – 1 softgel, twice daily. **Caution:** *Do not use if you take anticoagulants (blood thinners), are allergic to iodine, or if you will have surgery within a week.* Omega-3s (EFAs) fight inflammation that is often due to a reduction of estrogen.

Liquid Serotonin – Use 10 to 15 drops, under the tongue, twice daily, and at bedtime.

Carnitine – 500 mg capsule twice daily, morning and afternoon to reduce cholesterol, triglycerides while energizing your heart and muscles.

Mag Link – 1 to 2 tablets in the morning and 1 to 2 in the afternoon or evening OR use **Mag Chlor 90** – 10–20 drops in juice, 2 to 3 times daily. *If diarrhea or loose stools occur, take tablets or drops by spacing further apart or decrease dosage by 1.* Mag Link and Mag Chlor provides magnesium chloride, the same form of magnesium present in the body, so it is readily absorbed and tolerated.

DHEA – 1 capsule daily, (25 mg or 50 mg, depending on age) upon arising in morning. If you are taking HRT, consult with your physician before using. You should use either HRT or DHEA, but not both simultaneously. **Caution:** *Do not use if you have a history of cancer.*

PhytoBalance – 1 capsule, daily between meals. Phytobalance promotes healthy estrogen and progesterone activity while reducing hot flashes. PhytoBalance provides natural hormone balancing factors including, phytoestrogens, progesterone enhancers, and tonic herbs. Phytoestrogens are plants that contain estrogen-like substances that bind to estrogen receptors. PhytoBalance is a standardized herbal extract formula that provides comprehensive support for the body during the hormonal changes that occur during menopause. Both phytoestrogens and isoflavones mimic some of the effects of estrogen and may lower menopausal symptoms, risk of osteoporosis, hypertension and heart disease, and breast cancer. PhytoBalance contains black cohosh in the recommended amounts. Black cohosh helps relieve menopausal symptoms by establishing the body's natural balance with your organs and glands.

Progesterone Cream – If menopausal, 1 metered pump, twice daily of progesterone creme for 21 days, then off 7 days, and repeat. If you are PeriMenopause, use 1 pump, twice daily beginning the 12th day after menstrual flow starts and continue to day 27. Progesterone creme contains natural progesterone plus black cohosh. Using the pump version gives you 24 mg of progesterone and 20 mg of black cohosh. Progesterone opposes estrogen and helps the body breakdown estrogen and its metabolites so it can be removed. Progesterone helps to balance symptoms of estrogen dominance reducing symptoms of PMS. Progesterone may cause some sloughing of tissue. OR

Internal Harmony Cream – contains 25 mg natural progesterone and 2,000 I.U. of Vitamin D. Apply 1 full pump once daily to inner leg or arm, massaging well into the skin. If you are menstruating, apply once a day on days 12 through 27 of your cycle. (Period starts day 1.) If you are menopausal, apply once a day for 25 days followed by a 5 day break.

Cal Mag Zinc Complex capsules with Boron and Vitamin D – 3 capsules at bedtime.

Soy – 1 to 2 servings per day of either powder form or capsules form with isoflavones. Soy provides phytoestrogens helping to replace estrogen that drops at menopause. Eating or drinking soy also helps to elevate your estrogen levels.

Pumpkin Seed (Curbita) – 1 capsule three to four times a day for urinary incontinence or urgency. Pumpkin seed contains phytochemicals that help strengthen the muscles of the urinary tract enhancing the ability to hold urine in as well as totally empty the bladder. Clinical studies show that pumpkin seed oil reduces bladder pressure and improves the tone of the sphincter that opens and closes the urethra, thereby improving overall bladder health. Pumpkin seeds contain amino acids, phytosterols, minerals, fiber, EFAs, Vitamin E, carotenoids, and phytoestrogens.

If you are stressed out or anxious prior to meals, use **L–T,** 1 or 2 capsules, 30 minutes prior to eating to quiet your GI tract and reduce your stress OR use **Liquid Serotonin** 10 to 15 drops and ¼ capsule of **GABA 750** dissolved in 8 ounces of warm water. Stress causes a release of insulin and adrenaline that tightens up the digestive muscles, causing bloating. If this is a chronic condition, consider digestive enzymes such as **Super Pancreatin**.

Obsessive-Compulsive Disorder (OCD)

Anxious thoughts, or rituals, that you feel you cannot control, characterize obsessive-compulsive disorder (OCD). Persistent, unwelcome thoughts or images, and the urgent need to engage in certain rituals can plague you, if you have OCD.

You may be obsessed with germs, or dirt, so you wash your hands over and over. You can be filled with doubt, and feel the need to check things again and again. You might be preoccupied by thoughts of violence, and fear that people close to you will be harmed. You may spend long periods of time touching things or counting. Order or symmetry may preoccupy you. You may be worried by thoughts that are against your religious beliefs.

These disturbing thoughts or images are called obsessions. The rituals performed to prevent or dispel them are called compulsions. There is no pleasure in carrying out the rituals that you are drawn to—only temporary relief from the discomfort caused by the obsession.

Many healthy people can identify with having some

of the symptoms of OCD, such as checking the stove several times before leaving the house. But the disorder is usually diagnosed only when such activities consume at least an hour a day, prove very distressing, and interfere with daily life. Most adults with this condition recognize the senselessness of their condition, but they cannot stop. Although some people, especially children with OCD, may not realize their behavior is unusual. OCD strikes men and women in approximately equal numbers, and afflicts roughly 1 in 50 people. It can appear in childhood, adolescence, or adulthood, but usually starts in the teens or early adulthood. A third of adults with OCD experience their first symptoms as children. The course of the disease varies. Symptoms can come and go. They may ease over time, or they can grow progressively worse. Evidence suggests that OCD might run in families.

Depression or other anxiety disorders can accompany OCD. Some people with OCD have eating disorders. Additionally, they avoid situations in which they might have to confront their obsessions. They may try unsuccessfully to use alcohol or drugs to calm themselves. If the OCD grows severe enough, it can keep someone from holding down a job, or from carrying out normal responsibilities at home. Frequently, however, the disorder does not develop to those extremes.

Research by *National Institutes of Mental Health* scientists and other investigators led to the development of amino acid and behavioral treatments benefiting people with OCD. A combination of the treatments often benefits most patients. Some individuals respond best to one therapy, some to another. Behavioral therapy, specifically a type called exposure and response prevention, has also proven useful for treating OCD. It involves exposing the person to whatever triggers the problem, and then helping him or her forego the usual ritual. For instance, having the patient touch something dirty and then not washing his hands. This therapy succeeds in patients who complete a behavioral therapy program, although results have been less favorable in some people who have both OCD and depression. Address OCD and depression separately.

With OCD, as well as depression, research demonstrates that serotonin is involved in the biology of obsessive-compulsive behavior. As serotonin levels decrease, OCD behavior becomes more pervasive. Anxiety, depression, stress, especially post traumatic stress disorder and grief, use available serotonin. Those who suffer from OCD are victims of a serotonin–dopamine interaction gone wrong. Both serotonin and dopamine are the primary neurotransmitters in the brain's frontal lobes, where decisions are made. Neurotransmitters are the chemical agents responsible for transmitting impulses between nerve fibers, or from nerve fibers to a specific receptor. Using a balanced neurotransmitter complex, on a daily basis, along with 5-HTP, helps balance serotonin and dopamine levels.

Suggested Nutritional Support

Brain Link Complex – 3 scoops dissolved in juice, first thing in the morning OR use

T–L Vite – 1 capsule, in the morning.

Glutamine – 1,000 mg, in either capsules or powder, three times per day.

SBNC – 3 capsules in the morning and in the afternoon.

GABA 750 – ½ capsule dissolved in water, mid morning and mid afternoon.

Mood Sync – 1 or 2 capsules, twice to three times daily. Mood Sync combines 5-HTP, tyrosine, GABA, glutamine, taurine, and B6. **Caution:** *If you are taking an SSRI, SNRI, tricyclic, or MAOI antidepressant, or if you have a history or melanoma, do not use Mood Sync.* Instead use Anxiety Control 2 capsules, three times daily, plus L–T,®

1 to 2 capsules, three times daily along with SBNC and Neuro Links, 1 dropperful, twice to three times daily.

OR use **Tyrosine 850** – 1 in the morning, and 1 in the evening. If under 100 pounds, use tyrosine (500 mg), 1 in the morning and 1 in the evening. **Caution:** *Do not take tyrosine, if you are taking an SSRI, SNRI, tricyclic, or MAOI antidepressant, or if you have a history or melanoma.*

Liquid Serotonin – 10 to 15 drops, four times per day, or as needed.

Neuro Links – 1 dropperful up to four times daily as needed.

5-HTP – 2 capsules, 1 hour before bedtime. **Caution:** *Do not take tyrosine if you are taking an tricyclic, or MAOI antidepressant, or if you have a history or melanoma.*

Mag Link – 4 to 6 tablets per day, divided OR use

Mag Chlor 90 – 15–25 drops in juice, 2 to 3 times daily. *If diarrhea or loose stools occur, take tablets or drops by spacing further apart or decrease dosage by 1.*

B Complex Capsule – 1 capsule in the morning.

Methionine – 500 mg in the morning, and in the evening.

Probiotics (Acidophilus) – Eat some yogurt or kefir daily to boost good bacteria in the gut. Recent research shows a connection between the gut, the head, and behavior. Some research indicates that correction of gut bacteria can improve and even, eliminate mental disorders such as OCD.

Osteoarthritis

Age brings on constant change in the body, including degenerative joint changes or osteoarthritis. Osteoarthritis means inflammation of the joint that causes morning stiffness, pain, decreased range of motion, and in some cases deformity of the joint. Osteoarthritis affects 80% of individuals over the age of 50 with the most common joints affected are the knees, hips, spine, and hands. Most of the pain and inflammation results from normal wear and tear of everyday living. The joints that are used the most are the joints most often affected. However, food allergies can greatly accentuate the cartilage damage of the joints. Poor diet and deposition of minerals also contribute to the health of the joints. Additionally, emotional stress aggravates osteoarthritis. The old saying, "Mental stress brings physical illness," certainly applies to osteoarthritis. Increased stress increases muscle tension and poor posture stresses your joints. Stressed muscles pull on the joints thereby affecting the joint spaces. Overtime the stressed joints cause cartilage damage that contributes to the deterioration of the joint.

Other factors that can make osteoarthritis worse are food sensitivities (allergies) and weather. If you have environmental or other food allergies, they may be contributing to your joint aches and pain. You may be unaware that certain foods are aggravating your arthritis. Most common foods are the nightshades are called PPET or potatoes, pepper (bell), eggplants, tomatoes, and tobacco. But other common food allergies can inflame your joints that include wheat (breads, pasta), dairy products (milk, yogurt, ice cream), eggs, and beef. It is not uncommon to be allergic to the foods that you eat and crave the most.

But the real chore is identifying the foods that aggravate your arthritis. But if you change your diet, and drop the offending foods from your diet, you often experience less pain. Joint improvement is often seen in 2 to 6 weeks, but may take as long as 6 to 9 months. After 6 months, you may begin to slowly add the offending foods back in, if you find a particular food causes inflammation and pain, you have two choices, put up with the pain and swelling or drop the offending food(s) from your diet permanently.

When the weather changes, most commonly rain or

fall in barometric pressure, arthritis flare-ups are very common. Individuals with arthritis will tell you when the weather is going to change. It is as if their bones act as a barometer and forecast weather changes.

Glucosamine derives from glucose in the body and is the precursor to proteoglycans. Proteoglycans are a large group of protein substances found in the joint cartilage. The proteoglycans give the joint strength and resilience. Chondroitin sulfate (CS) is another substance that makes up the proteoglycan. CS exerts anti-inflammatory activity. Multiple studies showed that the combination of glucosamine and chondroitin are useful for arthritis.

Abram Hoffer in the 1950s found that niacinamide improved arthritis symptoms. The exact mechanism of action is unknown, but believed to be both anti-inflammatory, and as an analgesic. Niacinamide appears to help control the disease process itself. Benefits are usually seen at 3 to 4 weeks.

Fish oil is omega 3 fatty acids. Omega 3 fatty acids decrease inflammation including arthritis and other inflammatory conditions. Fish oil contains DHA or (docosahexaenoic acid) and EPA (eicosapentainoic acid). DHA is important in joint and brain health. EPA is an omega 3 that helps control inflammation in the body, the immune system, and blood clotting and circulation.

Vitamin C is important in collagen and proteoglycan formation. Low levels are connected to increased rates of osteoarthritis. Vitamin C provides the substances needed by the joints for repair and upkeep. Vitamin C is important for immunity and fights free radicals as it is an antioxidant.

Serrapeptase (SerraEnzyme) is an enzyme that is produced commercially in the lab through fermentation. Serrapepeptase helps to clear out inflammation and dead or scar tissues. This enables the body to heal itself by replacing or repairing the tissues involved. Overall, proteolytic enzymes like serrapeptase promote better movement, less thromboembolic complications, less pain and swelling, and less cartilage or capsular damage due to lack of movement.

Curcumin is an extract of Curcuma Longa, the biologically active part of turmeric. Curcumin usage stems back to Ayurvedic medicine that has been used for thousands of years. Over 500 references about curcumin and turmeric are available in peer-reviewed journals.

SAMe is the active form of methionine. SAMe works in many areas of the body, and has multiple benefits in different parts of the body. But SAMe is a fairly unstable compound that requires refrigeration. Utilizing methionine along with SBNC (Super Balanced Neurotransmitter Complex) instead derives the same benefits with less cost. The body uses the methionine to make as much SAMe as it needs. SAMe has anti-inflammatory, anti depressive, and repairs damage in joints. Studies show that SAMe worked as well as NSAIDS (Non Steroidal Anti-Inflammatory Drugs) with fewer side effects.

Suggested Nutritional Support

Glucosamine – Usual dosage is 1500 to 2,000 mg per day. Be patient as it may take 4 to 6 weeks for you to feel a difference with glucosamine. Conversely, if you quit taking glucosamine, it would continue to work for a month.

Chondroitin sulfate (CS) – usual dosage is 800- 1200 mg per day.

Niacinamide – Usual dosage is 1 to 3 grams of niacinamide per day. Some people experience nausea as a side effect from niacinamide. If this occurs, start with a lower dose, and take with food. Hepatotoxicity occurs in some people with high doses (over 1500 mg) of niacinamide daily.

Fish Oil – 3,000 to 4,000 mg per day.

MSM – 3,000 mg twice daily helps reduce joint pain and increased range of motion.

Vitamin D – 2,000 I.U. per day. If over the age of 60,

you need to double up on your dosage (take 4,000 I.U.) as you do not absorb as much as when you were younger. Vitamin D is important in the cartilage metabolism. Low levels of vitamin D are linked with more progression of osteoarthritis and incidence of the disease.

Easy C (Esterified C) with Bioflavonoids – 1000 mg, twice to three times per day

Methionine – 1500 mg, twice daily along with SBNC, 1 twice a day.

Serrapeptase (80,000 or 250,000 I.U.) – 1 to 3 (depending on finances) three times per day to start until symptoms lessen, then decrease to 1, twice a day.

Curcumin X 4000 – 1, twice to three times a day. To enhance uptake, use a curcumin that contains Meriva as this curcumin absorbs about 23 times greater than regular curcumin.

Panic Disorder

Panic disorder strikes at least 5.7% of the population, and is twice as common in women than in men. It can appear at any age, but most often it begins in young adults. Not everyone who experiences panic attacks will develop panic disorder. Many people have one attack, but never have another. If you do have panic disorder, it is important to seek treatment. If untreated, the disorder can become very disabling.

Panic often starts with anxiety. People with panic disorder experience sudden feelings of terror, repeatedly with no warning. While impossible to predict when an attack will occur, many develop intense anxiety between episodes, worrying when and where the next one will strike. In between times there is a persistent, lingering worry that another attack could come any minute.

When a panic attack strikes, your heart pounds, and

you feel sweaty, weak, faint, or dizzy. Your hands tingle or feel numb, and you feel flushed, or chilled. You can have chest pain or smothering sensations, a sense of unreality, fear of impending doom, or loss of control. You genuinely believe you are having a heart attack or stroke, losing your mind, or on the verge of death. Attacks can occur any time, even during non-dream sleep. While most attacks average a couple of minutes, occasionally they can go on for up to 20 minutes.

Often accompanied by other conditions such as depression or alcoholism, panic disorder may spawn phobias which can develop in places or situations where panic attacks have occurred. If a panic attack strikes while you are riding an elevator you can develop a fear of elevators, and start avoiding them.

Many people's lives become greatly restricted. You avoid normal, everyday activities such as grocery shopping, driving, or even leaving your home. You may be able to confront a feared situation only if accompanied by a spouse or other trusted person. Basically, you avoid

Panic Attack Symptoms

- Pounding heart
- Chest pains
- Light-headedness or dizziness
- Nausea or stomach problems
- Hot flushes or chills
- Tingling or numbness
- Shaking or trembling
- Feelings of unreality
- Shortness of breath
- Sensation of choking or smothering
- Tremors
- A feeling of being out of control or going crazy
- Fear of dying
- Sweating

any situation you fear might make you feel helpless if a panic attack occurs. When a person's life becomes so restricted by the disorder, as happens in approximately one third of all people with panic disorder, the condition is called agoraphobia. A tendency toward panic disorder and agoraphobia runs in families. Often, early treatment of panic disorder can stop the progression to agoraphobia.

Susan D. James on *ABC News' Good Morning America* reported that the gut could play a part in anxiety and other mental issues. Dr. James Greenblatt, a Boston psychiatrist, had a teenager with OCD, ADHD, and digestive problems. Dr. Greenblatt ordered a simple urine test for the metabolite HPHPA, a chemical by-product of clostridia bacteria. The teen's levels were elevated. He put her on probiotics to boost her good bacteria in her gut, and then a course of antibiotics. The teen's levels started to drop dramatically. After six months, the teen's symptoms began to disappear and by one year, all the symptoms were gone. Three years later, the teens had no sign of symptoms.

New research in the journal, *Science,* showed that fat and thin people have different bacteria in their gut. Could this lead to a different approach to weight loss? When the GI (gastrointestinal) health was changed and challenged for seniors in a nursing home, doctors used fecal transplant to improve mental health. Scientists now think there is a link between what is in the gut and what is in your head. Trillions of bacteria, in fact up to five pounds, resides in the average adult's digestive tract. Bacteria may participate more in disorders such as anxiety, schizophrenia, and autism. And who is to say, why it may also extend to other mental disorders?

Studies have shown proper treatment called cognitive behavioral therapy, orthomolecular therapy, or a combination of the two, helps 70 to 90% of people with panic disorder. Significant improvement occurs within

8 to 10 days.

The cognitive behavioral approach teaches you how to view the panic situations differently, and demonstrates ways to reduce anxiety by using breathing exercises or techniques to refocus your attention. Another technique used in cognitive behavioral therapy is called exposure therapy. This frequently helps alleviate the phobias resulting from panic disorder. In exposure therapy, you are very slowly exposed to the fearful situation a number of times until you become desensitized.

Most people find the greatest relief from panic disorder symptoms when they use orthomolecular therapy. Orthomolecular and cognitive behavioral therapies, can help relieve panic attacks and reduce their frequency.

Suggested Nutritional Support

Panic and anxiety can cause feelings of fatigue and loss of appetite. Nutrients taken daily in the morning are readily absorbed and give you a needed lift.

Brain Link Complex – Take in 8 ounces of fruit juice, and follow directions on can (dosage depends on weight).

Anxiety Control – 2 capsules, early morning, noon, and evening. Add 2 additional, if needed for panic OR use

GABA 750 – ½ capsule dissolved in water, mid morning. Repeat mid afternoon and evening. If under 125 pounds, use GABA 375 dissolved in water.

Liquid Serotonin – 10 to 15 drops, three times per day.

Neuro Links – 15 drops under the tongue, three to four times a day.

Mag Link – 2 tablets, twice to three times daily. Titrate to bowel tolerance. OR use

Mag Chlor 90 – 15–25 drops in juice, 2 to 3 times daily. If diarrhea or loose stools occur, take tablets or drops by spacing further apart or decrease dosage by 1.

Taurine 1000 – 1 capsule, twice daily.

5-HTP – 50 mg, an hour before bedtime. **Caution:** *If you are taking an SSRI, SNRI, tricyclic, or MAOI antidepressant, do not use 5-HTP* OR use

Sleep Link – 2 capsule (50 mg) an hour before bedtime, with juice. **Caution:** *If you are taking an SSRI, SNRI, tricyclic, or MAOI antidepressant, do not use Sleep Link or 5-HTP.* Instead use Anxiety Control, 2 capsules OR a 3 mg **Melatonin** capsule, 30 minutes before bed. You can combine the 5-HTP, Sleep Link, or Melatonin with Mag Chlor 90 to make a bedtime cocktail.

Mellow Mind (Ashwagandha) – 1 or 2 capsules at bedtime for sleep, if needed.

PoweRelief– 2 capsules, as needed for pain. Combine with Mag MAXX over the affected areas. **Caution:** *Do not use PoweRelief with DLPA if you have PKU, are pregnant or lactating, if you take MAO inhibitor or tricyclic antidepressants, or if you have a history of malignant melanoma.*

Periodontal Disease

Periodontal disease usually starts with gingivitis or inflamed gums. Inflamed gums are red, swollen, and bleed easily. Gingivitis usually results from a lack of brushing and tooth flossing that allows plague accumulation along the gum line of the teeth. Plague is a soft, sticky film that consists mainly of bacteria. Plague usually accumulates in faulty fillings, around the teeth, or next to poorly cleaned partials, bridges, etc. If the plague remains on the teeth more than 72 hours, it solidifies into tartar. Other conditions such as pregnancy, puberty, and birth control drugs are contributing factors to gingivitis.

Periodontal disease occurs when the gingivitis expands to the supporting structures of the teeth. Perodonitis occurs from extended accumulation of plague and tartar between the teeth and the gums. Pockets form between the tooth and the gum due to the gum irritation and become more inflamed. As the gums pull away from the tooth, a pocket forms and fills with more plague. Over time the plague harden and pockets become deeper and deeper extending into the root of the tooth. Eventually, plaque destroys the root of the tooth and the surrounding bone structure causing the tooth to loosen and fall out. The major cause of tooth loss in adults is periodontal disease. Certain medical conditions such as diabetes, Down's syndrome, Crohn's disease, low white blood cell levels, and AIDS, can make a person more vulnerable to periodontal disease.

Signs of periodontal disease include bleeding, red swollen gums, and bad breath (halitosis).

Suggested Nutritional Support

Mouthwash with Xylitol – rinse mouth, twice to four times a day, after brushing.

Easy C (Esterified C) – 2,000 mg, three times per day.

Coenzyme Q10 – 100 mg per day.

Borage Oil – 1,500 mg per day. Borage oil proved more effective than fish oil.

T–L Vite – 1 per day.

Folic Acid – 2 (800 mcg) twice daily. Folic acid helps decrease gingivitis.

Probiotics – daily intake of lactobacillus reuteri. This bacteria is most often found in children's yogurt.

Rain – Spray mouth as needed for dryness or to prevent tooth decay. Rain contains xylitol. **Warning:** *Do not let your pet get a hold of it as it will cause severe blood sugar drop that can be life-threatening.*

Spry – are xylitol flavored mints to prevent tooth decay and decrease bacteria in your mouth. **Warning:** *Do not let your pet get a hold of it as it will cause severe blood sugar drop that can be life-threatening.*

Premenstrual Syndrome (PMS)

Premenstrual Syndrome, or PMS, is a very distressing syndrome for many women. It commonly occurs in women of childbearing age, 7 to 10 days prior to onset of her period. The degree varies, but at least 50% of all women experience at least some symptoms of PMS. PMS bothers some women from the onset of menses, but most commonly, it affects women in the thirties and into the PeriMenopause years. In about half of these, the symptoms manifests so severely they need treatment or medical attention.

There are various risk factors for PMS. Research suggests that a hormone imbalance exists with PMS. Advancing age and the number of children increase the development of PMS. As a woman ages, the more painful periods experienced by women in their teens and twenties are often replaced by the appearance of PMS symptoms. The most severe and difficult cases of PMS are usually found in women in their forties. PMS symptoms usually start to overlap menopausal symptoms. The imbalance between progesterone and estrogen creates more symptoms of PMS and may be indicative of PeriMenopause.

Categories of PMS Symptoms

PMS A anxiety, nervous tension, mood swings, irritability

PMS B weight gain, swelling of breasts and extremities, breast tenderness, abdominal bloating

PMS C headache, increased appetite, cravings for sweets, fatigue, dizziness, fainting, pounding heart

PMS D depression, forgetfulness, crying, confusion, and insomnia

Suggested Nutritional Support

Rodex Forte (timed-release) – 1 capsule in the morning that contains B6 (150 mg), B12 (200 mcg), and folic acid (800 mcg).

Anxiety Control – For irritability and anxiety, use 2, three times per day.

Mood Sync – 1 or 2 capsules, twice to three times daily, as needed for mood swings and depression. **Caution:** *Do not use If you are taking an SSRI, SNRI, tricyclic, or MAOI antidepressant or have had a melanoma.*

Tyrosine 850 – For depression, 1 in the morning and 1 mid afternoon. **Caution:** *Do not use If you are taking an SSRI, SNRI, tricyclic, or MAOI antidepressant or have had a melanoma.*

Glycine – 1 or 2 capsules dissolved under tongue to cut sugar cravings.

Mag Link – 4 to 6 tablets per day, divided OR use

Mag Chlor 90 – 15–25 drops in juice, 2 to 3 times daily. *If diarrhea or loose stools occur, take tablets or drops by spacing further apart or decrease dosage by 1.* Magnesium is extremely important for many symptoms of PMS, including anxiety, painful menstruation, and headache prior to period. Magnesium helps with cramping and muscle spasms. Be patient with painful menstruation as it may take several months to increase your magnesium level.

PoweRelief – For pain relief, use 1 or 2 capsules, as needed. **Caution:** *Do not use PoweRelief that contains DLPA, if you have PKU. Do not use tyrosine if you take MAO inhibitor or tricyclic antidepressants, or if you have a history of a melanoma.*

T-L Vite – 1 capsule daily with main meal. T-L Vites are a combination multivitamin/mineral.

Glutamine – For memory and concentration, use 1 (500 mg) capsule, or ½ scoop glutamine powder, three times per day.

Chromium Picolinate – For sugar cravings and to help

stabilize blood sugar, use 1(200 mcg), twice per day.

5-HTP – For sleep and to balance the serotonin level, take 1 (50 mg) capsule 30 minutes before bedtime. **Caution:** *If you are taking an SSRI, SNRI, tricyclic, or MAOI antidepressant, do not use 5-HTP.*

Mellow Mind – 1 or 2 capsules, twice daily for stress. Ashwagandha in Mellow Mind increases serotonin.

Vitamin E – For breast tenderness, increase up to 2,000 I.U. a week before your period, then decrease and maintain with no more than 800 I.U. of Vitamin E per day.

Progesterone Cream (such as Internal Harmony Cream) – 1 pump applied to inner thigh or inner arm once daily. If you are menstruating, apply daily on days 12 to 27 of your cycle. Day 1 is when your period starts. Progesterone improves your mood and increases libido. Progesterone counterbalances the toxic effects of estrogen dominance.

DHEA – 1 (25 mg) upon arising in the morning, if you are over 40 years of age. **Caution:** *Do not use if you have a history of cancer.*

Pregnenolone – 10 to 50 mg upon arising in the morning, if you are over 40 years of age. **Caution:** *Do not use if you have a history of cancer.*

PhytoBalance – If you are over 40, you might consider this formula to offset your symptoms. Some of your symptoms may be PeriMenopause. This formula helps to balance your bouncing hormones.

Adrenal – 2 to 4 capsules as needed to help with stress.

Other Factors:
- Avoid caffeine (coffee), colas, and sugar to decrease anxiety, insomnia, nervousness. Colas and caffeine cause a loss of magnesium which amplify stress and anxiety.
- Avoid chocolate, and high intake of salt based foods, to decrease fluid retention and breast tenderness.
- Reduce or stop tobacco intake.
- Reduce the intake of fats; avoid fried foods and animal fats.

- Increase intake of fiber with complex carbohydrates, leafy vegetables, legumes, and fruits.
- Limit intake of alcohol, refined sugar, and red meat.
- Reduce stress through regular exercise. Use other stress-reduction techniques such as massage, meditation, and relaxation CDs.
- Eat yogurt, kefir, or take acidophilus supplements to boost your good bacteria in your gut. Research shows there is a connection between the gut and disorder in the head.

Post Traumatic Stress Disorder (PTSD)

Patients demonstrate symptoms of generalized anxiety and reoccurring flashbacks of traumatic episodes. PTSD usually occurs after a severe major stressor: fire, tornado, major auto accident, unexpected death, or military experience. Weeks or months after the traumatic episode occurs, flashbacks can begin and cause numerous physical symptoms such as sweating, rapid pulse, increased anxiety, panic, insomnia, and avoidance behaviors. Flashbacks can also cause a release of adrenaline. This sets stress reaction into high gear. Stress burns amino acids, and unless the brain is supplied with nourishment, it will continue to send anxiety-related messages that cause physical symptoms. A therapist experienced in PTSD and a good orthomolecular program will be helpful and aid the healing process.

PTSD is a debilitating condition that affects thousands of people. Often, people with PTSD have persistent frightening thoughts and memories of their ordeal, and feel emotionally numb. PTSD was once referred to as shell shock, or battle fatigue. It was first brought to public attention by war veterans. But, it can result from any number of traumatic incidents, serious accidents, natural disasters such as floods or earthquakes, or violent attacks such as mugging, rape, kidnapping, or torture. The event triggering the post trauma may be something that threatened the person's life, or the life of someone close to them, or it can be something they witnessed, such as the Oklahoma City bombing.

People with PTSD can relive the trauma in the form of nightmares, or disturbing recollections in which they experience the event over and over in their minds. They may also experience sleep problems, depression, feelings of detachment or numbness, or be easily startled. They may lose interest in things they once enjoyed, and have trouble showing affection. Sometimes, they feel more irritable or more aggressive than before the incident, and can even become violent. Memories that remind them of the incident can be very distressing, causing them to avoid certain places or situations that bring back to the event. Even anniversaries of the event are often very difficult.

PTSD can happen at any age. The disorder can be accompanied by anxiety, depression, or substance abuse. Symptoms may be mild or severe. People may become easily irritated or have violent outbursts. In severe cases they may have trouble working or socializing. In general, the symptoms seem to be worse if the event that triggered them was initiated by a person, such as a mugging or rape, as opposed to something like a flood.

Ordinary events can serve as reminders of the trauma and trigger flashbacks or intrusive memories. A flashback may make the person lose touch with reality and reenact the event for a period of seconds or hours, rarely days. A person having a flashback, which can come in the form of images, sounds, smells, or feelings, believes the traumatic incident is happening all over again.

Not every traumatized person gets full-blown PTSD, some don't experience PTSD at all. If the symptoms last more than a month, PTSD is the diagnosis. Symptoms usually occur within 3 months of the trauma, but the course of the illness varies. Some people recover within 6 months; others have symptoms that last much longer. The condition can become chronic. In some cases, PTSD may not arise until years after the traumatic event.

Amino acids can ease the symptoms of depression and sleep problems, but psychotherapy, especially cognitive behavioral therapy, is an integral part of treatment. Being exposed to a reminder of the trauma as part of the therapy, such as returning to the scene, sometimes helps. Support from family and friends can help speed recovery.

Antidepressants and tranquilizers only postpone healing and suppress symptoms. They do not restore the brain chemistry with needed nutrients.

Suggested Nutritional Support

S.B.N.C. – 2 capsules in the morning and afternoon.

Neuro Links – 15 drops under the tongue for acute episodes, and use 2 to 4 times daily, and if you awaken during the night.

Rodex Forte – 1 timed release capsule in the morning that contains B6 (150 mg), B12 (200 mcg), and folic acid (800 mcg).

T–L Vite (multivitamin) – 1 capsule, in the morning with breakfast.

Mag Link – 4 to 6 tablets per day, divided OR use

Mag Chlor 90 – 15–25 drops in juice, 2 to 3 times daily. *If diarrhea or loose stools occur, take tablets or drops by spacing further apart or decrease dosage by 1.*

Anxiety Control – 2 capsules, three times daily, for the first month after a traumatic episode, then 2 in the morning and 2 in the afternoon. Increase to 6 per day, if needed.

Easy C (Esterified C) – 1,000 mg, morning and evening.

PoweRelief – 2 capsules, twice daily, as needed for pain. As an alternative, use boswella, or DLPA. **Caution:** *Do not use PoweRelief or DLPA if you have PKU, are pregnant or lactating, if you take MAO inhibitor or tricyclic antidepressants, or if you have a history of melanoma.*

Mood Sync – If depression occurs, take 2 capsules, twice to three times daily. **Caution:** *If you are taking an SSRI, SNRI, tricyclic, or MAOI antidepressant, do not use Mood Sync.* Instead use Anxiety Control 2 capsules, three times daily, plus L–T,® 1 to 2 capsules, three times daily.

L–T – 2 capsules, twice to three times daily to keep your brain in a state of alpha (like deep meditation) without drowsiness.

5-HTP – 50 mg at bedtime. Take 2, if your sleep pattern is interrupted. **Caution:** *If you are taking an SSRI, SNRI, tricyclic, or MAOI antidepressant, do not use 5-HTP.*

Or use **Melatonin** – For sleep use 3 to 6 mg, an hour before bedtime. *If you have weird dreams or nightmares, reduce your dosage of melatonin.*

Probiotics (Acidophilus) – Take some acidophilus daily to boost good bacteria in the gut. Recent research shows a connection between the gut, the head, and behavior.

Other Factors

- Do not use alcohol in the acute stage of trauma.
- Decrease caffeine intake, and have none after noon.
- Limit sugar and soda intake.
- During the first month, avoid loud noises and bright lights.
- Use relaxation CDs, two to three times per week.

Post-Trauma Case History

Kelly is a 36-year old college professor who never had any major problems with anxiety or chronic pain until May 15, 1994. That day, while driving to the University, Kelly's life took a turn for the worse. She was hit broadside by a teenager. Her car was totaled, and so was her life.

Kelly spent a week in the hospital for painful neck and back injuries. Her healing was slow, and she had to learn to live with chronic pain and certain restrictions. But each day, Kelly improved a little more and tried to put her life back in order.

A few months passed without any particular problems. Then one day while driving to her classes, she heard a sound that she had hoped she would never hear again ... a car, unable to stop, slammed into the car in front of her. Kelly was not hurt, but she was so full of fear she had a full-blown panic attack. This was the beginning of her post traumatic stress disorder, and all the symptoms that go with it. As time went on, she began having flashbacks of her accident, and with the flashbacks came the physical symptoms. Kelly developed a dread of driving because she never knew when the flashbacks would occur. Her physical symptoms included palpitations, weakness, trembling, apprehensiveness, sweating, headaches, muscle spasms, and fear of dying. Kelly came in to see me. I explained post traumatic stress disorder and the symptoms. I started her on a relaxation program and nutritional supplements. She was totally depleted of neurotransmitters because of the chronic stress. Kelly's nutritional support program included Anxiety Control, Mag Link, PoweRelief, and B-complex. Within a few weeks she showed a marked improvement. Her headaches stopped, and her driving anxiety diminished. Post traumatic stress disorder can cause numerous psychological and physical problems, but with proper therapy, healing will occur.

Seasonal Affective Disorder (SAD)

Seasonal Affective Disorder, or SAD, is the only illness that demonstrates evidence of circadian rhythm disturbances. The symptoms of SAD occur only on a seasonal basis. Classical depression exhibits a daily rhythm that worsens in the morning and improves in the evening, with mood swings, and insomnia or disturbed sleep patterns. SAD symptoms always begin in autumn or early winter. SAD usually lasts five to seven months, until spring, when the days grow considerably longer, and the symptoms disappear. The person remains healthy until the following fall. Incidences of SAD increase almost proportionately to how far people live from the equator.

Four classic symptoms occur every fall and winter in most SAD sufferers:

- Increased desire to sleep
- Extreme lethargy
- Depression
- Increased appetite that often leads to weight gain

Melatonin greatly benefits SAD sufferers. Depression and melancholy are linked to a deficiency of neurotransmitters and neurohormones. Melatonin, taken nightly, supports the delicate brain balance.

The disruption of circadian rhythms can lead to stress-induced immunosuppression. Melatonin serves as an important anti-stress buffer. People with free-floating anxiety—anxiety without apparent cause—phobias, insomnia, and depression tend to have lower than

> **Direct Circadian Rhythm Influencers**
> - Sleep/wake cycle.
> - Neurotransmitters/neuropeptides.
> - Hormones.
> - Other factors such as age, mood changes, body temperature, blood pressure and pulse rate, jet lag.

normal levels of melatonin. Many of their symptoms ease after supplementing with melatonin. People with anxiety report marked improvement after adding melatonin and other inhibitory neurotransmitters.

Suggested Nutritional Support

Melatonin – 2 mg capsule, 30 minutes before bedtime. If you weigh over 200 pounds, use 3 to 6 mg of Melatonin to regulate your circadian rhythm. **Caution:** *Do not use if pregnant or lactating or less than 30 years old.*

DHEA – 25 mg capsule, first thing in the morning, on an empty stomach, if you are over 40. DHEA helps stressed adrenals. Consider having a DHEA sulfate level run to see exactly where your level is. By running the level prior

> **Drugs that Deplete Melatonin**
>
> **NSAIDs** (Non-Steroidal Anti-Inflammatory Drugs) such as aspirin, ibuprofen (Motrin), Lodeine, Orudis, Aleve, Dolobid.
>
> **Tranquilizers** such as Valium, Ativan.
>
> **Anti-anxiety** meds such as Xanax, Ativan, Prozac.
>
> **Calcium channel blockers** such as Cardizem, Procardia, Verapamil.
>
> **Beta blockers** such as Inderal, Lopressor, Tenormin.
>
> **Steroids** such as hydrocortisone, prednisone, Depo-Medrol.
>
> **Antidepressants** such as Prozac, Serzone, Effexor, Luvox.
>
> **Vitamin B12** in large doses.
>
> Source: Dr. Russel J. Reiter, University of Texas Health Science Center in San Antonio

to taking, you can see exactly how the DHEA is helping you. **Caution:** *Do not use if you have a history of cancer.*

Mood Sync – 1 or 2 capsules, twice daily, for stress and anxiety with depression. **Caution:** *If you are taking an SSRI, SNRI, tricyclic, or MAOI antidepressant, do not use Mood Sync.* Or use

HTP10– 2 capsules, twice daily. **Caution:** *If you are taking an SSRI, SNRI, tricyclic, or MAOI antidepressant, do not use 5-HTP* Or use

5-HTP – 1 to 2 (50 mg) capsule(s) in the morning, afternoon, and evening. 5-HTP is a direct precursor to serotonin, and it elevates your mood. If 50 mg of 5-HTP makes you sleepy, use the Mood Sync. **Caution:** *If you are taking an SSRI, SNRI, tricyclic, or MAOI antidepressant, do not use 5-HTP.*

Ginkgo – 40 mg, every morning. Ginkgo prevents metabolic and neural disturbances, and increases blood flow to the brain. **Caution:** *Stop using week prior to any anticipated surgery. Do not use if taking blood thinners.*

Mellow Mind – 1 (500 mg) capsule, twice daily, for adaptogenic influence on energy. **Caution:** *May cause blood sugar drop in diabetics.*

Other Factors

Light Therapy using full spectrum lights for ½ to 1 hour daily.

Teen Anger and Aggression
Neurotransmitter Deficiency

What makes some teenagers display angry and aggressive behavior, while others are calm and in control?

A growing number of scientists are looking at the delicate limbic system—the same area of the brain involved in ADD and ADHD. Research demonstrates alterations of function in the limbic system can cause changes in emotional responses like rage, fear, reasoning, and impulse control. The limbic system connects key parts of the brain such as the amygdala, hippocampus, and the cerebral cortex. All memories begin in the hippocampus, and all memories are stored in the amygdala. The limbic system marks all negative experiences for playback at a later time, especially experiences such as being abused as a child, or exposure to violent behavior. The teenage brain is immature and has not developed fully emotionally. Teens are impulsive and often fail to think through the consequences of their actions.

The environmental factor of growing up in a dysfunctional home causes teens to demonstrate aggressive behavior. But the majority of evidence gathered about aggressive behavior points to disturbed brain function and the overproduction of certain chemicals

Low Serotonin Deficiency Symptoms

- Aggression
- Depression
- Anxiety
- Panic attacks
- Mood swings
- Violent tendencies
- Hyperactivity
- Migraine headaches
- PMS syndrome
- Carbohydrate craving
- Insomnia
- Obesity
- Fibromyalgia
- Alchoholism
- Obsessive Compulsive Disorder
- Chronic pain

and the under production of others. Studies done at the University of Illinois Medical School found children and teens, with aggressive and disruptive behavior, all had low levels of the major inhibitory neurotransmitter, serotonin. Serotonin levels most accurately predict how teens and children will react to punishment. Serotonin transmits electrical impulses in the brain from one neuron to another. Low levels of serotonin interrupt the smooth transmission of impulses, and the brain receives mixed signals. According to Ronald Kotulak, author of *Inside the Brain,* scientists now believe that, along with the nation's increase in violence, low serotonin may be responsible for a steady increase in depression, especially among children.

Blood tests done on one hundred teens and children at the Pain & Stress Center reflect major deficiencies of neurotransmitters. When the deficiencies were corrected with amino acid supplementation, behavior problems ranging from aggression, anger, ADD, ADHD, behavioral disorders, poor concentration, and depression, all diminished remarkably. Inborn metabolic errors, chronic stress and anxiety, as well as overconsumption of junk food, caffeine, sugar, and alcohol, can cause neurotransmitter deficiencies. And chronic stress burnout can kill brain cells.

Scientists have also reported a tendency for aggression can be inherited and found in aggressive genes. This predisposes a teen to anger, violence, and depression, and this gene could be passed on to his or her children. Children who have an alcoholic parent can inherit the alcoholic gene, and demonstrate the same amino acid deficiencies that cause the craving for alcohol. GABA and glutamine, two major neurotransmitters, shut off the craving switch in the brain. When the brain chemistry is in balance, impulsive and aggressive behavior patterns do not dominate brain function.

Serotonin enables impulses in the brain to

harmonize. Serotonin-producing cells send out over five hundred thousand connections to cells in every part of the brain. Serotonin is the only neurotransmitter able to do that. For teens, the best serotonin source is 5-HTP, or 5-Hydroxytryptophan. The formula, Teen Link, is specially formulated for the teen's brain. Teen Link contains 5-HTP, GABA, glutamine, tyrosine, taurine, and Vitamins B6 and C.

There is no one solution to teen anger and violence. In addition to supplementing children's diets with amino acids, parents should consider counseling sessions with a behavior therapist for their children. Behavior therapists are trained in talk therapy and can help troubled teens sort out their feelings, and feel better about themselves. The longer negative feelings stay buried, the more powerful they become. This brain activity not only uses all available neurotransmitters, it also sets up a chain reaction that causes a teen to withdraw and allow his or her problems to go unresolved.

Drugs do not create new and needed neurotransmitters. Parents mistakenly put their children on Prozac, Zoloft, Serzone, or other drugs, to elevate their children's serotonin levels. These drugs only use available neurotransmitters. Drugs do not create new needed neurotransmitters. Drugs only mask symptoms and repress anger that should be resolved. There are neurotransmitter formulas available that can be given to children and teens safely, without the possibility of addiction or side effects.

The brain produces the only chemicals you will ever need. The key is to correct neurotransmitter imbalances in the brain and control aggression by adjusting brain levels of serotonin. Available serotonin declines in situations where chronic stress controls a person's life. Impulsive and angry behavior becomes a way of life, setting the stage for possible violent behavior. The teen's brain never slows down, and must be provided on a daily basis with proper nourishment in the form of balanced neurotransmitters. A complete neurotransmitter formula should contain the amino acids: glutamine, GABA, taurine, phenylalanine, glycine, arginine, methionine, valine, lysine, leucine, alanine, isoleucine, histidine, and pyridoxal 5'phosphate (B6) to activate the amino acids.

Suggested Nutritional Support

T-L Vite – 1 capsule with main meal. T-L Vite is a high quality multivitamin/mineral OR use

Brain Link Complex – 2 scoops in the morning in fruit juice.

SBNC (Super Balanced Neurotransmitter Complex) – 2 capsules in the morning; if over 150 pounds, use 3 capsules.

Mag Link – 4 to 6 tablets per day, divided OR use

Mag Chlor 90 – 15–25 drops in juice, 2 to 3 times daily. *If diarrhea or loose stools occur, space tablets or drops further apart or decrease dosage by 1.*

Lysine – 500 mg capsule, twice to three times daily for facial or body skin problem, or herpes.

Anxiety Control – 1 or 2 capsules, twice to three times daily for stress and anxiety.

Teen Link – 1 capsule in the morning, and in the afternoon. If over 125 pounds, use 2 capsules. **Caution:** *Do not use If you are taking an SSRI, SNRI, tricyclic, or MAOI antidepressant or have had a melanoma.*

Cal Mag Zinc Complex with Vitamin D and Boron – 2 capsules, at bedtime. If over 150 pounds, use 3 capsules.

5-HTP – 1 to 2 (50 mg) capsules at bedtime OR use

Sleep Link – 1 to 2 capsule (50 mg) an hour before bedtime, with juice. If needed, add a 500 mg Mellow Mind (Ashwagandha). **Caution:** *If you are taking an SSRI, SNRI, tricyclic, or MAOI antidepressant, do not use Sleep Link or 5-HTP.* Instead use Anxiety Control, 2 capsules OR Mellow Mind, 30 minutes before bed.

Probiotics (Acidophilus) – Take some daily to boost good bacteria in the gut. Recent research shows a connection between the gut, the head, and behavior.

Tourette's Syndrome

In the 1960s, the medical profession recognized Tourette's Syndrome to be among the most-pervasive movement disorders. Over the years, more cases were studied and clinical researchers began to accumulate results of studies from large groups of clients. Agreement was reached that the base symptoms of multiple motor and vocal tics were onset in childhood.

Over the past five to ten years, many changes occurred in the diagnosis and understanding of Tourette's Syndrome. The most significant is the relationship of Tourette's Syndrome to other tic disorders. Continued research demonstrated the association of behavior problems, especially attention deficit disorder, hyperactivity, and obsessive-compulsive disorder.

The clinical criteria for Tourette's Syndrome include the presence of multiple motor tics, vocal tics, and behavioral problems, as well as environmental context. The onset of Tourette's occurs between the ages of two and thirteen, and can intermittently worsen, especially during times of high stress, emotional tension, or stimulant use.

Simple motor tics are abrupt, brief, isolated movements such as eye blinks, head twitches, shoulder shrugs, or facial grimaces. The vocal tics include a variety of inarticulate noises and sounds, such as throat clearing, sniffing, grunting, and groaning. Tics may manifest themselves by virtually any body movement, noise, or certain nutrient deficiencies. According to Roger Kurlan, M.D., Department of Neurology, University of Rochester School of Medicine, some problems found in school-age children with Tourette's

Syndrome include:

- Motor tics, phonic tics, and mental energy expended in suppressing tics
- Obsessive-Compulsive behaviors
- Attention Deficit Disorder with hyperactivity
- School and other phobias, test anxiety, conduct disorder, or depression
- Short temper or argumentative
- Associated learning disabilities
- Poor social skills
- Low self-esteem
- Medication side effects

Gerald Golden, M.D., Director, Child Development Center and Professor of Pediatrics, Department of Neurology, University of Texas, published a paper in the July 1988 *Psychiatric Annals*, on the relationship between stimulant medication and tics. Dr. Golden states "all of the stimulant drugs commonly used to treat attention deficit disorder have been reported to increase tic response. Tourette's was precipitated by treatment with Ritalin, Dexedrine, and Cylert. Similar responses has been reported with the use of Imipramine." His report reflects clinical evidence that supports the observation that stimulant drugs increase the severity of tics 25 to 50% in patients with Tourette's, and occasionally can precipitate Tourette's Syndrome in a patient who did not previously manifest symptoms of this disorder. Researchers concluded that obsessive-compulsive disorder can coexist with Tourette's Syndrome. It now appears that there is a genetic link for those with OCD and Tourette's Syndrome. If the family already has a history of multiple chemical sensitivities, the potential for children to display the symptoms increases.

Sherry Rogers, M.D., author of *Tired or Toxic?*, reports the tics of Tourette's Syndrome represent abnormal "firings" of the nervous system. According to Dr. Rogers, the study of Tourette's Syndrome individuals can represent the entire field of environmental medicine and nutritional biochemistry. Some common mineral abnormalities, such as magnesium deficiency, can exist. Many individuals can have hidden food sensitivities, and dust, inhalants, and mold sensitivities. In her book, Dr. Rogers addresses the possibilities of environmental factors first, and then proceeds with a treatment program which has proven very successful. All the research points to evidence that Tourette's Syndrome can have multiple triggers, and those who present with the symptoms should be evaluated to establish the underlying causes. Patients treated with prescription medication(s) do not improve, and side effects from the medication can aggravate the symptoms and increase depression and a feeling of hopelessness.

Doris Rapp, M.D., author of *Is This Your Child's World?*, feels physicians should explore all aspects to determine the primary cause of Tourette's Syndrome, and that prescription drugs are certainly not the answer. Dr. Rapp suggests starting by eliminating toxic chemicals from the diet and environment: caffeine, foods, dust, molds and pollens. Exposure to certain chemicals such as gas, paint, or pesticides, can cause Tourette's Syndrome symptoms to become more overt. What is important is for parents to recognize what triggers Tourette's Syndrome symptoms in the first place. Caution should be taken by those who have Tourette's Syndrome to avoid commonly suspected triggers such as cigarette smoke, pesticides, perfumed products, animal hair, alcohol, dust, and areas with high-mold counts. After eliminating exposure to these chemicals, you will notice positive behavior changes and increased motor skills in people with Tourette's.

Suggested Nutritional Support

Brain Link – Add to your favorite fruit juice, according to weight. Brain Link Complex is a total neurotransmitter complex, in powder form, for children; or for adults, if you prefer a drink formula. If you prefer a capsule, use 1 **T-L Vite**, along with 2 **SBNC (Super Balanced Neurotransmitter** Complex) capsules. Teens can use either the Brain Link or the T-L Vite, plus the SBNC caps.

Folic Acid – Add 1 (400 mcg) daily. Folic acid is important for neurological functioning.

Easy C (Esterified C) – Children under 100 pounds, use 1,000 mg, daily. Adults use 1,000 mg, three times daily.

Mag Link – 4 to 6 tablets per day, divided OR use

Mag Chlor 90 – 15–25 drops in juice, 2 to 3 times daily. *If diarrhea or loose stools occur, take tablets or drops by spacing further apart or decrease dosage by 1.* For children, use Calcium Magnesium Liquid – It has a peppermint taste. Follow the instructions on the bottle OR Mag Chlor 90 – 5 to 12 drops in juice, 2 to three times daily.

L-T – 2 capsules, three times daily OR use

Anxiety Control – 1 or 2 capsules, as needed to reduce stress and anxiety. Teens use 1 or 2 **Teen Link**. Children under 50 pounds, use an extra scoop of Brain Link.

Vitamin E – Adults use 800 I.U. of Vitamin E; teens and children use only 400 I.U.; if a child weighs less than 50 pounds, use 200 I.U. Use Vitamin E to improve symptoms of neurological dysfunction.

Neuro Links – ½ dropper; use as needed, daily, for children and adults.

5-HTP– 50 mg capsule 30 minutes before bed for adults. If sleep problems persist, use 2 capsules. Teens, use 50 mg of **5-HTP** capsule OR 1 to 3 **HTP10** capsules. Children, use 1 to 2 HTP10 capsules, 30 minutes prior to bedtime. **Caution:** *Do not use if you are taking a SSRI, SNRI, tricyclic, or MAOI antidepressant or have had a melanoma.*

Taurine 1000 – 1 (1000 mg) capsule, three times daily. For children, use 500 mg, three times daily.

Vinpocetine – 1 capsule in the morning, in adults, or if over 100 pounds (**Caution:** *If pregnant or lactating, do not use.*) OR use

Huperzine – 1 capsule twice daily for memory and concentration. **Caution:** *Do not use if you are a pregnant or lactating woman, or if you have heart, pulmonary, or asthma problems.*

HTP10 – Children with Tourette's, ADD/ADHD, need additional neurotransmitters for school. HTP10 is a low-dose 5-HTP for children, or small adults. Use 1 HTP10 in the morning, and 1 after lunch, to help children stay on task and focus, or for excessive movement. **Caution:** *Do not use if you are taking a SSRI, SNRI, tricyclic, or MAOI antidepressant, or have had a melanoma.*

Probiotics – Give your child some yogurt (appropriate for age) to support immune system and gut-head connection.

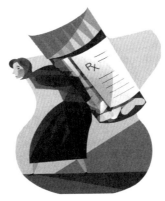

Prescription drugs do not put nutrients back into the brain and body. Rather, it robs your nutrients. The key is to put back in the brain what belongs there—nutrients—amino acids, vitamins, and minerals!

Amino Acid Testing

The body constantly conducts many complicated series of chemical reactions in precisely controlled ways to keep us healthy. Over 5,000 reactions occur every second in a cell. By utilizing the natural substances in optimal quantities to reestablish a normal balance, you can help correct the cause of some disease processes in a nontoxic way.

Amino acid metabolism disorders are becoming recognized as a major factor in many disease processes. Amino acid analysis is an analytical technique on the leading edge of nutritional biochemical medicine. It gives a new approach toward illness, and assists patients who have not responded to treatment as expected, or who present complex cases with diverse symptoms.

Amino acid analysis of urine or plasma goes a long way toward assessing vitamin and mineral sta-

---

Amino Acid Analysis Has Proven Helpful With

- Chronic fatigue
- Candida infections
- Food and chemical sensitivities
- Immune system disorders
- Anxiety
- Depression
- Learning disorders
- ADD/Hyperactivity
- Behavioral disorders
- Eating disorders
- Cancer
- Hypoglycemia
- Diabetes
- Cardiovascular disease
- Seizures
- Headaches
- Arthritis
- Chronic pain

tus. Amino acid analysis measures the levels of amino acids in the body that affect many important processes. Additionally, it provides insights into the patient's functional needs for a wide variety of vitamins and minerals. Many of the enzymes which catalyze the interconversion of amino acids require vitamin and mineral cofactors to function optimally. In many cases where incomplete conversion of one reaction to another is due to sluggish enzymes, this indicates a functional need for increasing levels of a cofactor.

Food Allergy Profile

Food allergies are a common problem for people who have addiction tendencies or dependence. The test reports over 100 foods, sensitivity rating, and gives you a complete diet to follow.

Essential Fatty Acid Profile

EFAs are vital to brain function, correcting mood disorders, depression, and gastrointestinal problems. The test provides a guide to the EFAs and the amounts needed by the brain.

Comprehensive Vitamin Profile

This profile provides a complete analysis of 17 vitamins and specific amounts needed by your brain and body. This test helps establish your deficiency problems.

DHEA Sulfate Level

DHEA is the Mother Hormone because it is the precursor of all steroid hormones including estrogen, testosterone, and cortisol. Aging, stress, pain, depression, anxiety, and certain diseases cause your DHEA level to drop drastically. The drop in DHEA compounds your body's ability to respond to stresses, diseases, and makes you age more rapidly. If you are over 40, you should have your DHEA level checked. Consider adding DHEA to your supplement program first thing in the morning if you are over 40. DHEA is available in capsule form or in a transdermal cream. *But do not use DHEA if you have had cancer.*

Testing?

For detailed information about these tests and pricing, call the Pain & Stress Management Clinic at (800) 669-2256 Monday through Friday.

General Summary of Amino Acids

In order to absorb and assimilate *any amino acid*, you must take B6 or P5'P daily. The other important co-factor is magnesium. Magnesium is a facilitator, and is involved in over 300 enzyme reactions in the body.

ALANINE

- Nonessential amino acid.
- Functions as a neurotransmitter and found in high concentrations in the brain
- Alternate source of glucose for the liver
- May play a role in prostate health and reduce BPH symptoms in combination with glycine and glutamic acid

Therapeutic dosages: 200 to 800 mg per day

ARGININE

- An essential amino acid
- Helps in treatment of burns, elevated ammonia levels, and cirrhosis of the liver by detoxifying ammonia
- Stimulates immune response by enhancing the production of T cells
- Induces growth hormone release from the pituitary gland
- Intake should be kept low in herpes simplex and Epstein Barr virus interactions
- Required for normal sperm count
- Enhances fat metabolism
- Stimulates immune system, muscle growth, fat metabolism, muscle relaxation, and sexual enhancement

- Promotes vasodilation with increased blood flow to heart arteries
- Prevents blood clotting without increasing risk of stroke, GI bleed, or kidney damage.
- Acts as a neurotransmitter in the brain playing a role in learning and memory
- NO *Should be used with caution in schizophrenics*

Therapeutic dosages: Up to 10,000 mg per day, divided

ASPARTIC ACID

- Nonessential amino acid and major excitatory neurotransmitter
- Protective function over the liver
- Promotes mineral uptake in intestinal tract
- Helps with metabolism of ammonia and other toxins
- Acts to transport magnesium and potassium to the cells
- Metabolizes carbohydrates via the Krebs cycle and forms parts of DNA and RNA
- Energy source for the body
- Stimulates the thymus gland, antibody formation, and immune system
- Increases amino acids such as GABA in the brain when given with arginine

CARNITINE

- Nonessential amino acid composed of methionine and lysine in the body
- Found primarily in the muscles
- Helps lower triglycerides, cholesterol, and increase HDL levels
- Essential in transportation of long chain fatty acids into the cells where fats are converted into energy

- In heart disease and angina patients improves oxygen usage and metabolism of energy while increases exercise endurance
- Increases muscle strength and exercise tolerance
- Reduces left ventricular and diastolic pressures
- In uremia or kidney disease, may reduce risk factor for atherosclerosis and coronary heart disease
- Helps with depression
- Vegans at higher risk for deficiencies

Therapeutic dosages: 1,000 to 4,000 mg per day

ACETYL-L-CARNITINE
- Subcategory of carnitine
- Readily crosses blood brain barrier
- Improves mental clarity and focus with slight mood elevation
- Protects brain against oxidation and prevents brain cell degeneration
- Stimulates acetylcholine for memory and helps brain cells connect and communicate
- Delays progression of Alzheimer's in younger patients

Therapeutic dosages: 1,000 mg twice daily. Up to 4,000 mg per day with dementias.

CITRULLINE
- Produces the amino acids, Arginine and Ornithine
- Detoxifies ammonia or other *nitrogen* waste products
- Product of nitric acid formation from arginine
- Stimulates growth hormone production

CYSTEINE
- Derived from serine and methionine in the liver

- A major sulfur containing amino acid.
- Serves as an alternative energy source
- Helps maintain skin flexibility and texture by slowing abnormal cross linking of collagen
- Acts as an antioxidant that prevents free radical formation
- Useful in iron deficiency, anemia and promotion of iron absorption
- Promotes red and white blood cell reproduction and tissue restoration in lung diseases
- Converts to cystine in lack of Vitamin C
- Heavy metal chelator
- Helps protect against effects of alcohol, pollution, and cigarette smoke
- Assists in prevention of cataracts
- A derivative called NAC is helpful with asthma, bronchitis and sinus drainage by liquefying and thinning mucus
- NAC helps in preventing side effects and damage from chemo and radiation therapies
- Studies demonstrate that NAC reduces artery clogging (vascular cell adhesion molecule or VCAM-1 activity) with 1,200 mg per day while increasing glutathione
- Do not use in large amounts in diabetics due to changes in insulin activity, but diabetics need more cysteine and taurine than average person

Therapeutic dosages: 250 to 600 mg twice to three times daily

CYSTINE

- Nonessential amino acid formed by combining two cysteine compounds.

- Chief sulfur containing compound in protein and helps give proteins their shape
- Least soluble of all of the naturally occurring amino acids
- Helps enhance the immune system by increasing white blood cell activity
- Helpful with psoriasis and eczema
- Important for skin flexibility and texture and along with cysteine is necessary for collagen health
- Enhances tissue recovery after surgery
- Part of insulin molecule
- High content in hair
- Proven to protect the body—brain and liver against damage from alcohol and cigarette smoking.
- Use with caution in people predisposed to stone formation in the liver or kidneys
- *Do not use large amounts if diabetic.* Diabetics using insulin as cystine inactivates insulin by reducing certain compounds.

GABA (GAMMA AMINO BUTYRIC ACID)
- Reduces anxiety/stress by decreasing limbic firing
- Helps decrease muscular tension due to stress
- Assists with hyperactivity and ADD
- Crosses blood brain-barrier

Therapeutic dosages: 600 to 3000 mg per day, divided

GLUTAMIC ACID
- Principle excitatory neurotransmitter in the brain and most abundant in the CNS.
- Essential for the removal of ammonia from the brain and transportation of potassium to the brain

- Critical for proper cell function and essential in metabolic rate processes.
- Controls gastric function.
- Source of energy for mucosa
- Promotes bone formation
- Encourages glutathione production.
- Component of glucose tolerance factor
- Helpful with muscular dystrophy and other neurological conditions such as Parkinson's and epilepsy
- Useful in maintaining the body's nitrogen balance

GLUTAMINE

- Conditionally essential amino acid and most important amino acid in the blood
- Derives from histidine and glutamic acid
- Serves as chief energy source for many body tissues
- Functions as a precursor and an inhibitor of nitric oxide formation
- Helps with acid-base balance
- Principle route of nitrogen removal from skeletal muscles
- Helps with ulcer and intestinal healing and digestion
- Helps protect body from effects of alcohol
- Assists in treatment of alcoholism by decreasing the desire to drink
- Crosses blood-brain-barrier
- Aids mental functions such as memory and concentration and acts as energy source in the brain
- Helps decrease intestinal permeability from food allergies
- Assists in muscle growth and repairs
- Needed for production of other nonessential amino acids

- Enhances effectiveness of chemotherapy and radiation treatments for cancer, while reducing toxicity and damage to the body

Therapeutic dosages: 500 to 4000 mg per day, divided

GLUTATHIONE

- Composed of cysteine, glycine, and glutamate
- Important for DNA synthesis and repair
- Is an antioxidant that reduces free radical damage
- Antitoxin that neutralizes exogenous stressors and negative lifestyles such as air pollution, smoking, petrochemicals, chemicals, pesticides, and chlorine
- Enzyme cofactor and activation
- Protective effect against radiation therapy, and acts as a reductant for drugs and chemicals
- Enhances immune system
- Transports other amino acids into the cell

Therapeutic dosages: 1000 to 3000 mg per day, divided

GLYCINE

- Nonessential and simplest amino acid
- Has sweet taste and readily dissolves in liquids
- Inhibitory neurotransmitter
- Helps with anxiety and hyperactivity
- Helps to remove lead from the body
- Assists with epilepsy
- Low levels reported in ALS

Therapeutic dosages: 500 to 3000 mg per day, divided.

HISTIDINE

- Essential amino acids for infants, not adults

- Helps relieve pain due to rheumatoid arthritis
- Should always be taken with Vitamin C (Esterified C such as Easy C)
- Use with caution in females prone to depression from P.M.S.
- Mild anti-inflammatory effect
- Metabolized into the neurotransmitter histamine that is involved in smooth muscle function in blood vessels
- Helps maintain the myelin sheath or insulator of certain nerves
- Necessary for proper functioning of auditory nerves
- Chelates toxic metals from the body
- Helpful with nausea during pregnancy
- High levels seen with OCD, depression, and phobias
- Low levels seen with rheumatoid arthritis and Parkinson's disease
- Precursor for histamine

Therapeutic dosages: 1000 to 6000 mg per day

ISOLEUCINE

- One of the Branched Chain Amino Acids, and should be taken as a group. BCAAs are present in 70% of all bodily proteins
- Plays a role in blood sugar regulation and low levels result in hypoglycemia-like symptoms
- Required for the formation of hemoglobin
- Enhances energy, endurance and assists in muscle tissue repairs
- Important in post-operative, burn and trauma patients to prevent muscle wasting
- Very low levels seen in chronic renal failure patients
- Adults require 12 mg per kilogram (kg) of body weight daily; children ages 10 to 12 require 29 mg per kg; infants 80 mg per kg

Therapeutic dosages: 250 to 700 mg per day. Best as BCAA group supplement.

LEUCINE

- Second of the Branched Chain Amino Acids, and should be taken as a group
- Found in large quantities in the muscles
- Great producer of energy under many kinds of stress from trauma to surgery, infection, muscle training, and weight lifting
- Only amino acid that can substitute for glucose while fasting
- Promotes insulin production and release that stimulates protein synthesis and inhibits protein breakdown
- Increases re-utilization of other amino acids in multiple organs
- Helps with blood sugar regulation
- Helps with Parkinson's disease in large doses
- Use with all kinds of stress
- Helps in the growth and repair of vital tissues and production of growth hormone
- Adults require 16 mg per kilogram (kg) of body weight daily; children ages 10 to 12 require 42 mg per kg; infants 128 mg per kg

Therapeutic dosages: BCAA as a group, use 175 to 1200 mg per day.

LYSINE

- Essential amino acid that is found in large amounts in muscle, connective, and collagen tissues
- Inhibits growth and replication of herpes (Type I and II) and Epstein Barr viruses

- Promotes growth, especially bone growth in infants and children, both requiring much larger amounts in adults
- Required for antibody formation
- Helps with lead toxicity
- Tends to be low in vegetarians
- Precursor to carnitine, and its formation
- Stimulates calcium absorption
- Encourages growth and repair of muscles
- Involved in development and management of collagen, antibody formation, enzyme and hormone development

Therapeutic dosages: 1000 to 3000 mg per day with Vitamin C, divided

METHIONINE
- An essential sulfur-containing amino acid
- Powerful antioxidant and detoxifies the liver
- Converts to glutathione that helps neutralize chemicals and toxins
- Key component associated with many essential physiological processes.
- Detoxifies heavy metals from the body and excessive levels of histamine
- Involved in synthesis of choline and adrenaline, lecithin, and Vitamin B12
- Always take with B6 to inhibit synthesis of homocysteine that promotes plague deposits in arteries. Homocysteine is produced from the metabolism of methionine
- Necessary so selenium is available to the body

Therapeutic dosages: 800 to 3000 mg per day, divided

ORNITHINE
- May reduce fat and increase muscle mass
- Powerful stimulator of growth hormone production by pituitary gland
- Assists in detoxification of ammonia in urea cycle
- Stimulates immune system and enhances wound healing
- May be useful in autoimmune disease such as arthritis
- Can be converted in body to arginine, glutamine, or proline
- Doses of 1000 mg in some people may cause insomnia
- Vital for body building tissues

Therapeutic dosages: 500 to 3000 mg per day, divided

PHENYLALANINE
- A precursor of the catecholamines, epinephrine, norepinephrine, dopamine and dopa
- May be helpful with appetite control by stimulating CCK (choleocystokinin enzyme).
- Increases blood pressure in hypotension

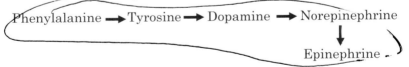

Phenylalanine → Tyrosine → Dopamine → Norepinephrine → Epinephrine

Note: *Should not be taken with MAOI and tricyclic antidepressants, with a history of cancerous melanoma, or if PKU (phenylketonuria) is present*

Therapeutic dosages: 500 to 2000 mg per day, divided

PROLINE
- Helps lower blood pressure
- Important in muscle, tendon and collagen repairs

General Summary of Amino Acids / 241

- Assists in skin flexibility in relation to aging and sun exposure, and essential for skin health
- A major amino acid in collagen if Vitamin C is present

Therapeutic dosages: 500 to 1000 mg per day with Vitamin C

TAURINE

- Conditionally essential amino acid
- Manufactured in the body from methionine and cysteine in the liver with B6. Some zinc must be present in body for taurine to function properly
- Found in foods of animal origin and one of the sulfur amino acids. Highest concentrations found in the neutrophil and the retina while the largest collection is found in the skeletal and cardiac muscles
- Predominant amino acid found in heart and assists in balancing calcium and potassium in the heart
- Under stress, more taurine is used in the body
- Useful in Congestive Heart Failure patients by easing their physical signs and symptoms *without side effects. Combine with CoEnzyme Q10 for most beneficial results.*
- Increases left ventricular heart performance without changes in blood pressure
- Low levels are associated with retinal (eye) degeneration and in diabetics, especially insulin dependent diabetics. Domestic pets, cats and dogs, tend to have low levels since commercial dog foods lack taurine.
- Helps with seizures and epilepsy that modulates nerve excitability
- Detoxifier of secondary bile acids and toxin
- Stabilizes and protects cell membranes
- Frequently considered a neuromodulator. Low levels may contribute to memory loss or Alzheimer's disease.

- Influences blood glucose and insulin levels effectively alleviating some of the complications of Type I (insulin dependent) diabetes and reducing platelet aggregation (platelet clumping for clot formation)
- Zinc enhances taurine's effect
- Helps decrease pain in chronic pain sufferers
- Decreases severity of steatorrhea (fatty stools) associated with cystic fibrosis with 30 mg per kg taurine supplementation
- For acute alcohol withdrawal psychotic episodes, use 1 gram three times daily for 7 days

Therapeutic dosages: 500 to 3,000 mg per day, divided. Certain conditions require doses up to 6,000 mg per day.

THEANINE

- A new amino acid that derives from green tea, but is not found in the human body
- Induces an alpha state in the brain *without drowsiness* in 40 minutes or less.
- Promotes formation of GABA in the brain and readily crosses the blood-brain-barrier
- Assists with anxiety and stress by increasing serotonin, dopamine, and GABA
- Lowers blood pressure
- Increases focus, concentration, and learning
- Reduces tension and muscle pain
- Modulates mood as theanine has a significant effect on neurotransmitter release of dopamine and serotonin
- Counters effects of caffeine

Therapeutic dosages for adults: 100 to 200 mg, three to four times daily

Therapeutic dosages for children 50 to 100 mg, twice daily for children over 6 years of age

THREONINE

- An essential amino acid; threonine rises three times normal during pregnancy
- Vital part of many proteins including collagen, elastin, and tooth enamel
- Important in development and support of the thymus gland, neurotransmitter production, overall health of the nervous system
- Only essential amino acid that can convert to glycine and serine for detoxification support
- Immune system supports and stimulates formation of antibodies. Threonine levels decrease with age and increase during times of stress or severe trauma
- Necessary for digestive and intestinal function
- Critical for liver health and plays a role in preventing accumulation of fat in liver
- Increases glycine levels in brain, and noticeably reduces ALS symptoms, treatment of MS, other nervous system diseases, and depression
- Reduces leg muscles spasms
- Cuts detoxification demands, especially glutathione
- Essential for mental health

Therapeutic dosages: 100 to 1,200 mg per day. In some cases of depression it requires 1,000 mg of threonine, twice daily.

TRYPTOPHAN (5-HTP or 5-hydroxytryptophan)

- An essential amino acid and neurotransmitter
- Precursor to serotonin and melatonin
- Neurohormone found in organs throughout the body
- Precursor of niacin, and effective in treating pellagra
- Appears to assist in blood clotting mechanisms
- Helps with insomnia in doses of 500 to 2000 mg

- Helps in depression and schizophrenia
- Useful in weight control
- Helps with pain by elevating the pain threshold
- Acts as mood stabilizer—calms aggression, OCD, violent and mania behaviors
- Take with B6 with carbohydrates such as fruit juice for maximum uptake to brain
- Helps decrease tremors in Parkinson's patients

Note: Tryptophan or 5-HTP should not be taken with SSRIs (Selective Serotonin Reuptake Inhibitors such as Prozac, Paxil, Luvox, or Effexor; SNRI (Serotonin Norepinephrine Reuptake Inhibitor) MAOI, or tricyclic antidepressants.

Therapeutic dosages: 5-HTP 50 to 100 mg day divided

Tryptophan → 5-HTP → Serotonin

5-HTP is about 10 times stronger than tryptophan, and is only one step biochemically away from serotonin.

Normal tryptophan dose is 500 to 4000 mg per day, divided

TYROSINE

- Nonessential amino acid that derives from phenylalanine and is precursor to catecholamines, epinephrine, norepinephrine, dopamine and dopa
- Precursor of thyroid hormones
- Assists in normal brain function and supplier of neurotransmitters
- Can be used in place of many antidepressants
- Helps stabilize blood pressure
- Involved in tissue pigmentation (melanin)
- Often called the *Stress* amino acid

- May improve memory, concentration, and alertness.
- Useful in people with Parkinson's disease

Note: *Should not be taken with MAOI and tricyclic antidepressants, and if you have a history of melanoma*

Therapeutic dosages: 500 to 2000 mg per day, divided

VALINE

- Third of the Branched Chain Amino Acids, that should be taken as a group, and an essential amino acid needed for the nitrogen balance in the body
- Necessary for muscle coordination, mental and neural function
- Helpful with inflammation
- Adults require 14 mg per kilogram (kg) of body weight daily; children ages 10 to 12 require 25 mg per kg; infants 89 mg per kg

Therapeutic Dosage: up to 1000 mg daily. Best if taken as BCAA

Research from UCLA demonstrates if the brain of a fifty-year-old person could be fully emptied of all impressions and memories it has stored and recorded on tape, the length of the tape would reach to the moon and back several times.

Food Sources of Some Amino Acids

Alanine: yeast, spirulina, seaweed (kelp), sesame seeds, soy, fish, beef, gelatins, wheat germ, turkey, duck, cottage cheese, and sausage.

Arginine: carob, chocolate, cabbage, cottage cheese, cheese, poultry, meats, fish, beans, grains, nuts and seeds, gelatin, cereals (especially buckwheat, oatmeal, and millet), soy, milk, eggs, wheat germ, vegetables (especially green peas, asparagus, broccoli, swiss chard, corn, potatoes, onion, spinach), brown rice, seeds, popcorn, grains, avocados.

Aspartic Acid: seaweed (kelp), sesame seeds, soy, meats such as pork, turkey, sausage, chicken, eggs, fish, gelatins, wheat germ, cottage and ricotta cheese.

Cysteine: meat, chicken, turkey, fish, grains, beans (especially soy), eggs, nuts, seeds, milk, cheese, cereals, couscous wheat.

Cystine: lentils, seeds, soy, beef, pork, buffalo, eggs, oat bran, seaweed (kelp), fish, chicken, veal, horseradish, milk, Tabasco sauce, safflower seeds, coffee, asparagus.

Glycine: seaweed (kelp) and spirulina, crustaceans, ostrich, pork, lamb, buffalo, beef, gelatins, veal, soy, fish, turkey, watercress, sunflower seeds, spinach, egg whites, chicken, turnips.

Histidine: meats, game meats such as deer, pheasant, chicken, turkey, fish, beans (especially soy), cheese, cottage cheese, pork, milk, eggs, grains, nuts, seeds, cereals, potatoes.

Isoleucine: chicken, turkey, meats, fish, beans (especially soy), milk, cheese, eggs, grains, cereals (especially millet), nuts, seeds, vegetables including swiss chard, corn, green peas, potatoes, spinach, avocado.

Leucine: chicken, turkey, fish, beans, milk, meats, cheese, eggs, grains, cereals (especially millet), nuts, seeds, gelatin, vegetables including sweet potatoes, potatoes, spinach, corn, green peas, asparagus, broccoli, swiss chard, mushrooms, tomatoes, avocado, wheat germ.

Food Sources of Some Amino Acids / 247

Lysine: yeast, parsley, soy, beef, cheese, chicken, turkey, meats, beans, dairy including milk, cheese, eggs, grains, cereals (especially oatmeal), gelatin, vegetables including potatoes, green peas, asparagus, broccoli, corn, mushrooms, spinach, avocado, wheat germ, chocolate.

Methionine: fish, turkey, chicken, crustaceans, cottage cheese, game meats such as elk or moose, buffalo, seeds, seaweed (kelp), spirulina, beans, nuts, seeds, cereals (especially millet, couscous and oatmeal), gelatin.

Phenylalanine: seaweed spirulina, watercress, chicken, turkey, meats, fish, daily including milk and cheese, crustaceans, egg whites, beans, grains, cereals (especially millet and oatmeal), nuts, seeds, vegetables including sweet potatoes, potatoes, spinach, corn, green peas, asparagus, swiss chard, gelatin, avocado, chocolate.

Proline: soy, cabbage, bamboo shoots, cottage, Parmesan, ricotta, and other cheeses, ostrich, beef, chicken, yogurt, gelatins, fish, milk, egg whites, pork, turkey, seaweed, spinach asparagus, soy sauce, horseradish, parley, kidney beans.

Serine: eggs, turkey, seaweed, spirulina, soy, fish, crustaceans, cottage cheese, pork, gelatin, game meat, kidney beans, sunflower seeds, veal.

Taurine: meat, poultry, eggs, dairy products, fish.

Theanine: green tea.

Threonine: water cress, seaweed (kelp), soy, fish, chicken, turkey, meats, beans, dairy including milk and cheeses, egg whites, beef, grains, nuts, seeds, cereals, gelatin, some vegetables including corn, green peas, potatoes, spinach, and cabbage.

Tryptophan: spinach, seaweed (kelp), watercress, mushrooms, soy, crustaceans, chicken, turkey, pork, meats, beans, dairy including milk and cheeses, grains, cereals, nuts, seeds.

Tyrosine: chicken, turkey, pork, beef, fish, beans, dairy including milk and cheeses, cereals (especially oatmeal and couscous), some vegetables including corn, potatoes, spinach, nuts, seeds

Valine: chicken, turkey, pork, beef, fish, dairy including milk and cheeses, cereals (especially millet, buckwheat, oatmeal), some vegetables including potatoes, sweet potatoes, broccoli, corn, green peas, spinach, swiss chard, avocado, chocolate..

Quick Reference

The following provides at a glance reference for specific conditions. Everybody's needs are unique and some nutrients may work better for you than others. For specifics including amounts, go to the appropriate section in this book. *Please review cautions below to assure you are using the supplements correctly to minimize possible drug-supplement interactions and side effects.*

CAUTIONS

Do not use essential fatty acids such as fish oil or ProDHA if you take anticoagulants (blood thinners), anticipate surgery within a week, or have an iodine allergy.

Do not use Huperzine if you have pulmonary problems, asthma, have congestive heart disease, or are pregnant or lactating.

Do not use phenylalanine if you have PKU, pregnant or lactating, have a history of melanoma, cancer, or use MAOI or tricyclic antidepressants.

Do not use Mood Sync, Teen Link, 5-HTP, tyrosine, HTP10, or Sleep Link if you are taking a SSRI, SNRI, MAOI, or tricyclic antidepressant.

Do not use phenylalanine, DLPA, or PoweRelief capsules if you have PKU, pregnant or lactating, have a history of melanoma, or use MAOI or tricyclic antidepressants.

Do not use lithium if you are pregnant, lactating, have cardiovascular disease, or use ACE inhibitors.

Do not use ginkgo if you take an anticoagulant (blood thinner). Use extreme caution if you take anti-inflammatory medications such as Motrin, pregnant, lactating, or have diabetes.

Anti-Aging

Nutritional support includes methionine, 5-HTP, glutamine, Esterified Vitamin C, SBNC, melatonin, Coenzyme Q10, Vitamin E, Huperzine A, antioxidants, flax, decaffeinated green tea extract, ProDHA or fish oil, digestive enzymes such as Pancreatin 650, magnesium chloride (Mag Link or Mag Chlor), DHEA, Pregnenolone, NAC, fiber, organic fruits and vegetables.

Avoid chemicals and pesticides.

Aggressiveness

Nutritional support includes 5-HTP, GABA, glycine, glutamine, taurine, tyrosine, or formula such as Mood Sync or Teen Link, B6 (timed-release), Neuro Links, fish oil, and probiotics.

Avoid phenylalanine, sugar, caffeine.

Alzheimer's Disease

Nutritional support includes SBNC, glutamine, ginkgo, B6 (timed-release), acetyl-l-carnitine (ALC), Esterified Vitamin C, phosphatidylserine, Huperzine A, EFAs such as fish oil or ProDHA, B12 injections, DHEA, Mag Link or Mag Chlor, decaf green tea extract, GalantaMind.

Avoid processed foods, alcohol, cigarette smoke, pesticides, and the minerals, aluminum and mercury.

Arthritis (Osteo)

Nutritional support includes histidine, cysteine, SBNC, boswella, glucosamine, chondroitin, Malic Acid Plus, DLPA, Esterified Vitamin C, magnesium (Mag Link), MSM, Serrapeptase, curcumin, beta glucan.

Avoid nightshade foods (PPET)—peppers, potatoes, eggplant, and tomatoes, processed foods, dairy products, and red meat.

Autism
Nutritional support includes Brain Link Complex, HTP10, B6 or P5'P, 5-HTP, glutamine, magnesium, Neuro Links, ProDHA (adults), DHA, Jr. (children), and probiotics.

Body Building
Nutritional support includes BCAA, alanine, arginine, carnitine, ornithine, Alpha KG, decaf green tea extract.

Cancer
Nutritional support includes NAC, taurine, glutamine, SBNC, Esterified Vitamin C, antioxidants, BCAA, melatonin, Brain Link Complex, flax, beta glucan, green tea extract (decaf), DIMM, BioDim D-Ribose, probiotics.

Avoid phenylalanine and tyrosine with history of melanoma, pesticides and chemical exposures.

For a detailed program on cancer, refer to *Definitive Guide to Cancer* by W. John Diamond, M.D., et al.

Cholesterol
Nutritional support includes carnitine, methionine, arginine, glycine, taurine, chromium picolinate, fortified flax, CoEnzyme Q10, EFAs such as fish oil, fiber, garlic, red yeast rice.

Avoid saturated fats. Use monounsaturated fats such as olive or canola oils. Eat whole grains, lean meats and fish, and complex carbohydrates. Be aware many anti-cholesterol drugs (statins) lower your CoQ10 levels, putting you at greater risk for a heart attack or a stroke.

Chronic Illness
Nutritional support includes BCAA, SBNC, NAC for cysteine, glutamine, 5-HTP, Esterified Vitamin C, antioxidants, L–T (Theanine with GABA & Glycine), T–L Vites or Brain Link Complex, green tea extract (decaf), probiotics. Increase organic fruit and vegetables and natural meats.

Avoid pesticides and chemicals.

Chronic Pain

Nutritional support includes 5-HTP, DLPA, GABA, glutamine, SBNC, boswella, magnesium (Mag Link or Mag Chlor), Esterified Vitamin C, PoweRelief, Serrapeptase, Curcumin, Mag MAXX Cream, and probiotics.

Avoid pain medications as you buildup a tolerance and require more drugs to get relief. Many pain medications are addictive.

Depression

Nutritional support includes 5-HTP, phenylalanine, tyrosine, SBNC, methionine, GABA, carnitine, threonine, taurine, Mood Sync, Rodex Forte, EFAs such fish oil, Mag Link or Mag Chlor, probiotics.

Avoid arginine. Use extreme caution if combining with antidepressant medications. See specifics in this book or talk with a pharmacist.

Diabetes

Nutritional support includes 5-HTP, carnitine, taurine, chromium picolinate, Mag Link (magnesium chloride capsules or Mag Link liquid), Esterified Vitamin C, Vitamin E, vanadium, alpha lipoic acid, blood sugar balance, bitter melon, green tea extract, gymnema sylvestre, EFAs such as fish oil, probiotics.

Avoid simple sugars and carbohydrates. Use complex carbohydrates, whole grains, lean meats, low fat diet, and many vegetables with low carbs or starches.

Drug Addiction

Nutritional support includes GABA, SBNC, tyrosine, glutamine, methionine, DLPA, B-complex, 5-HTP, Rodex Forte B6 (timed-release), Mood Sync, Anxiety Control or L–T. Read *Break Your Prescribed Addiction.*

Avoid alcohol and drugs.

Energy

Nutritional support includes carnitine, tyrosine or phenylalanine, CoQ10, Alpha KG, decaffeinated green tea extract, D-Ribose. If over 40, consider supplementing with DHEA 25 to 50 mg and/or Pregnenolone, probiotics.

Avoid food (sensitivities or allergies) that causes fatigue.

Epilepsy

Nutritional support includes glycine, GABA, taurine, B6, melatonin, 5-HTP, L–T.

Avoid strobe lights, pesticides, and chemicals.

Gallbladder

Nutritional support includes taurine, methionine, glycine, BCAA, digestive enzymes, pancreatin, probiotics.

Avoid fatty foods.

Heart Failure

Nutritional support includes taurine, tyrosine, carnitine, BCAA, CoEnzyme Q10, Mag Link (magnesium chloride tablets) or Mag Chlor liquid, L–T, decaffeinated green tea extract.

Hepatitis C

Nutrients support includes alpha lipoic acid, selenium, Silymarin, B-complex, decaf green tea extract, NAC, Esterified Vitamin C, Vitamin E, CoQ10, T–L Vites, EFAs such as ProDHA or fish oil. Use Anxiety Control, L–T, or Mood Sync to keep stress down. Use high fiber whole grain diet with organic fruits and vegetables.

Avoid smoking, alcohol, acetaminophen (Tylenol), food additive, mycotoxins, and general anesthesia.

Nutritional support includes lysine, Esterified Vitamin C, Vitamin B-complex, Vitamin E, Vitamin B12 injectable while in blister state, PoweRelief, DLPA, Beta Glucan, (L–T, Mood Sync or Anxiety Control).

Avoid arginine.

Hyperactivity

Nutritional support includes GABA, glycine, glutamine, taurine, Brain Link Complex, 5-HTP, Liquid Serotonin, SBNC, HTP10, Mood Sync or Teen Link or L–T, Neuro Links, probiotics.

Hypertension

Nutritional support includes 5-HTP, GABA, taurine, SBNC, Mag Link (magnesium chloride tablets) or Mag Chlor liquid, calcium, CoEnzyme Q10, Anxiety Control or Mood Sync, arginine, L–T, decaf green tea extract. *Avoid stimulants, caffeine, anger, and emotional upsets.*

Hypoglycemia

Nutritional support includes alanine, GABA, chromium picolinate, vanadium, Mag Link (magnesium chloride tablets) or Mag Chlor liquid, gymnema sylvestre, alpha lipoic acid. Eat small frequent, high protein meals. *Avoid high glycemic index carbohydrates.* Instead use low to mid glycemic index foods to help stabilize blood sugar.

Insomnia

Nutritional support includes 5-HTP, melatonin, GABA, Mood Sync, Mag Link (magnesium chloride tablets) or Mag Chlor liquid, Sleep Link, Neuro Links. Combine Mag Chlor with L-T for a bedtime cocktail. Use relaxation CDs such as *Relax by the Sea* to help relax and sleep. *Avoid phenylalanine.*

Leg Ulcers

Nutritional support includes cysteine such as NAC, glycine, threonine, BCAA, Esterified Vitamin C, zinc, Mag Link (magnesium chloride or Mag Chlor).

Liver Disease

Nutritional support includes alpha lipoic acid, selenium, silymarin, BCAA, carnitine, glutamine, B6.

Mania

Nutritional support includes SBNC, 5-HTP, GABA, glycine, SBNC, glutamine, Mood Sync, natural lithium, probiotics.
Avoid phenylalanine, tyrosine, and stimulants.

Memory/Concentration

Nutritional support includes glutamine, GABA, ginkgo, Huperzine A, Acetyl-L-Carnitine, SBNC, B6 (timed-release), Vinpocetine, Phosphatidylserine, galantamine such as GalantaMind.

Mental Alertness

Nutritional support includes tyrosine, phenylalanine, glutamine, ginkgo, Huperzine A, Vinpocetine, Phosphatidylserine, NeuroLinks, ALC (acetyl-l-carnitine), D-ribose.

Parkinson's Disease

Nutritional support includes phenylalanine, tyrosine, taurine, SBNC, 5-HTP, methionine, Mag Link (magnesium chloride capsules) or Mag Chlor, Esterified Vitamin C.

Radiation

Nutritional support includes NAC, glutamine, taurine, Esterified Vitamin C, beta-carotene, antioxidants, green tea extract, DIMM, BioDim, iodine, D-Ribose, probiotics.

Renal Failure

Nutritional support includes SBNC, carnitine, BCAA.

Schizophrenia

Nutritional support includes GABA, isoleucine, 5-HTP, methionine, B6, non-flush niacin, galantamine (GalantaMind), probiotics.
Avoid serine, leucine, asparagine. Check for food allergies.

Seizures

Nutritional support includes glycine, GABA, taurine, B6, melatonin, 5-HTP, L–T, Mag Link.

Avoid strobe or flashing lights, pesticides, and chemicals.

Stress

Nutritional support includes Anxiety Control, tyrosine, GABA, SBNC, Mood Sync, glutamine, glycine, histidine, Mellow Mind, Esterified Vitamin C, Mag Link (magnesium chloride tablets or Mag Chlor liquid), probiotics.

Avoid sugar, caffeine in all forms.

Surgery

Nutritional support includes BCAA, SBNC, glutamine, Esterified Vitamin C, beta-carotene, Beta Glucan, decaf green tea extract, Brain Link Complex, NAC, L–T or Anxiety Control, probiotics.

Avoid herbs and EFAs such as fish oil prior to surgery for at least 1 week.

Tardive Dyskinesia

Nutritional support includes GABA, taurine, BCAA, glutamine, Mag Link (magnesium chloride) or Mag Chlor liquid, L–T.

Tobacco Addiction

Nutritional support includes tyrosine, GABA, 5-HTP, glutamine, methionine, B Complex, Posinol, Mood Sync.

Avoid trying to stop more than one addiction at a time. Do not try to stop drinking caffeine at the same time you are trying to stop smoking.

Weight Control

Nutritional support includes 5-HTP, phenylalanine, GABA, tyrosine, SBNC, Mood Sync, probiotics. Eat whole grain, low carbohydrate diet with lean meats and an *abundance of vegetables and fresh fruits.*

Drug-Nutrient Actions

Drug/Condition	Supports	Depleted by
Anticonvulsants	Taurine, GABA, Glycine, 5-HTP, and Magnesium	Aspartic Acid
Antidepressants	Phenylalanine, Tyrosine, Methionine, Taurine, Theanine, EFAs.	Glycine, Histidine
Heart Failure	Taurine, CoQ10, Carnitine, Magnesium, Arginine,	Niacin, 5-HTP
Hypertension	Magnesium, Arginine, CoQ10, GABA, Theanine	
High Cholesterol	Carnitine, Magnesium, EFAs, Red Yeast Rice Chromium Picolinate	Cholesterol lowering drugs depletes magnesium and Vitamin D
Triglycerides	Chromium Picolinate, Carnitine	Glutamic Acid
Anabolic Steroids	BCAA, Carnitine	Arginine
Viral Antagonists	Lysine, Zinc	

Product Information

The *purity* of amino acids and nutritional supplements is very important to your success. Be selective. Your body responds to what you absorb. Absorption enhances when you *use only pharmaceutical-grade products.*

There are four grades of supplemental amino acids and nutritional products. We list them in order of purity from least pure to purest:

- Food lot
- Cosmetic
- Pharmaceutical grade
- I.V. grade

Pharmaceutical grade generally guarantees purity of product. Capsules are generally cleaner and purer than tablets, and *more bioavailable.* Tablets require fillers and binders. When considering nutritional supplements, look for preservative-free and excipient-free products because they are better. Buy supplements that are free of preservatives, fillers, binders, or excipients of any kind. *Insist on pharmaceutical-grade products. Your body and brain will know the difference.*

For information on products and other books, call 1-800-669-2256 or visit Pain & Stress Center website: http://www.painstresscenter.com

The mind suffers... the body cries...
the brain starves...

Bibliography

Aatron Medical Services, Inc. *Amino Acids Metabolism and Analysis.* 1989.

Adair, J.C. J.E. Knoefel, and N. Morgan. "Controlled trial of N-acetylcysteine for patients with probable Alzheimer's disease." *Neurology,* Vol. 57, No. 8, 2001, pp. 1515–1517.

Alschler, Lise. "Gymnema sylvestre's impact on blood sugar levels." *American Journal of Natural Medicine.* Vol. 5, No. 9, November 1998, pp. 28–30.

Amaducci L., et al. "Use of phosphatidylserine in Alzheimer's Disease." *Annuals New York Academy of Science.* Vol. 640, 1991, pp. 245–249.

Ang-Lee, Michael K, J. Moss, C.S. Yuan. "Herbal medicines and perioperatve care." *JAMA,* 2001, pp. 208–216.

Askanazi J., Y.A. Carpenter, C.B. Michelsen, et al. "Muscle and plasma amino acids following injury: Influence of intercurrent infection." *Annuals of Surgery,* Vol. 192, 1980; pp. 78–85.

Askanazi, J., D.H. Elwyn, J.M. Kinney, et al. "Muscle and plasma amino acids after injury: The role of inactivity." *Annuals of Surgery.* Vol. 188, 1978, pp. 797–803.

Babal, Ken. "The Fall and Rise of Tryptophan," *Nutrition Science News,* February, 1998, Vol. 3, No. 2, pp. 60–64.

Balch, James F. and Phyllis Balch. *Prescription for Nutritional Healing.* Garden City Park, NY: Avery Publishing Group, 1997.

Balch, James, and Mark Stengler. *Prescription for Natural Cures.* Hoboken, NJ: John Wiley & Sons. 2004. pp. 54–59, 537.

Barbeau, A. *Archives of Neurology.* Vol. 30, 1982, pp. 52–58.

Barbeau, Andre and Ryan J. Huxtable. *Taurine.* New York, NY: Raven Press, 1975.

Barbeau, Andre and Ryan J. Huxtable. *Taurine and Neurological Disorders.* New York, NY: Raven Press, 1978.

Berkow, Robert, Editor in Chief. *The Merck Manual of Diagnosis and Therapy.* 14th Ed. Vol. 1. 1982, pp. 954–964.

Berkow, Robert, Ed. T*he Merck Manual of Medical Information.* Whitehouse Station, NJ: Merck Research Laboratories, 1997, pp. 467–470.

Berkow, Robert, Ed. The Merck Manual of Medical Information. Whitehouse Station, NJ: Merck Research Laboratories, 1997, pp. 467–470.

Berkson, Burton M. "Practical Approaches to the Treatment of Acute and Chronic Liver Disease." 12th Intl. Symp. on Functional Medicine, May 26–28, 2005. *The Immune System Under Siege*, pp. 249–291.

Biolo, G., G. Toigo, B. Ciocchi, et al. "Metabolic response to injury and sepsis: changes in protein metabolism." *Nutrition.* Vol. 13, 1997, pp. S52-S57.

Bipolar disorder. *National Institute of Mental Health.* http://www.nimh.nih.gov/health/publications/bipolar-disorder/complete-index.shtml

Birdsall, Timothy C. "Therapeutic Applications of Taurine." *Alternative Medicine Review.* Vol. 3, No. 2, 1998, pp. 128–136.

Bland, Jeffrey, Ed. *Medical Applications of Clinical Nutrition.* New Canaan, CT: Keats Publishing, 1983.

Bland, Jeffrey S. Psychoneuro-Nutritional Medicine: An Advancing Paradigm. *Alternative Therapies.* May, 1995, pp. 22–27.

Block, K.O. and M. Friedman. *Absorption and Utilization of Amino Acids.* Boca Raton: CRC Press, Volume 1, 1989.

Block, Melissa L. "Improved Urinary Tract Health with Pumpkin Seed Extract." *The Doctor's Prescription for Healthy Living.* Vol. 9, No. 7, p. 13.

Bliznakov, and Gerald L. Hunt. *The Miracle Nutrient: CoEnzyme Q10.* New York: Bantam Books, 1987, pp. 65–123.

Blomstrand, E., S. Ek, and E.A. Newsholme. "Influence of ingesting a solution of branched-chain amino on plasma and muscle concentrations of amino acids during prolonged submaximal exercise." *Nutrition,* Vol. 12 1996, pp.485–490.

Blumenthal M, A. Goldberg A, J. Brinckman, Eds. *Herbal Medicine: Expanded Commission E Monographs.* Integrative Medicine Communication, 1999.

Bowery, N.G., et al. (ed.) *GABAB Receptors in Mammalian Function.* New York: John Wiley & Sons, 1990. *Brain Research Bulletin.* Vol. 48, pp. 203–209.

Bralley, J. Alexander and Richard S. Lord, Eds. *Laboratory Evaluations in Nutritional Medicine.* June/October 1999, pp. 4–19.

Braverman, Eric and Carl C. Pfeiffer. *The Healing Nutrients Within.* New Canaan, CT: Keats Publishing, Inc., 1987.

Breggin, Peter. *Talking Back to Ritalin.* Monroe, ME: Common Courage Press, 1998.

Breggin, Peter. *Toxic Psychiatry.* New York: St. Martin's Press, 1991.

Brittenden J, et al. 1994. Natural cytotoxicity in breast cancer patients receiving neoadjuvant chemotherapy: effects of L-arginine supplementation. *Eur J Surg Oncol* 20:467-72.

Broker, P. et al. "A two centre, randomized, double-blind trial of ornithine oxoglutarate in 194 elderly, ambulatory, convalescent subjects." *Age Aging.* Vol. 23, 1994, pp. 303–306.

Brown, R.P., P.L. Gerbarg, and T. Bottiglieri. "Adenosylmethionine in the clinical practice of psychiatry, neurology, and internal medicine." *Clinical Practice Internal Medicine,* Vol. 1, 2000, pp. 230–241.

Brownstein, David. Exploring the Controveries in Iodine Supplementation to Safely Improve Thyroid Function: Holistic Medicine for 21st Centrury. Institute for Functional Medicine 14th International Symposium, Tuscon, AZ May 23–26, 2007, pp. 433-487.

Bucci, L. J.F. Hickson, J.M. Pivarnik, et al. "Ornithine ingestion and growth hormone release in bodybuilders." *Nutrition Research,* Vol. 10, 1990, pp. 239–245.

"Carnitine: A Science behind a Conditionally Essential Nutrient Conference." NIH: Office of Dietary Supplements, March 25–26, 2004.

Carter, Rita. *Mapping the Mind.* Berkeley, CA: University of California Press, 1998, p. 23.

Cenacchi T. et al. "Cognitive decline in the elderly: A double-bind, placebo-controlled multicenter study on efficacy of phosphatidylserine administration." *Aging Clinical Experimental Research.* Vol. 5. 1993, pp. 123–133.

Chaitow, Leon. *Thorsons Guide to Amino Acids.* London: Thorsons, 1991.
Chen, L.H. "Biomedical Influences on Nutrition of the Elderly." *Nutritional Aspects of Aging.* Boca Raton: CRC Press, 1986.
Chetlin, Robert D. et al. "The Effect of Ornithine Alpha-Ketoglutarate (Okg) on Healthy, Weight Trained Men." *Journal of Exercise Physiology* online. Vol. 3, No. 4, 2000.
Citivelli, R. et al. "Dietary L-Lysine and calcium metabolism in humans." *Nutrition,* Vol. 8 1992, pp. 400–404.
Cohn, Suzy. *Drug Muggers.* Rodale, 2011, pp. 174–176, 229–239.
Cooper, Jack R., et al. *The Biochemical Basis of Neuropharmacology.* New York: Oxford University Press, 1990.
Coudray-Lucas, C. H. LeBever, L. Cynober, et al. "Ornithine alpha-ketoglutarate improves wound healing in severe burn patients: a prospective randomized double blind versus isonitrogensous controls.*Critical Care Medicine.* Vol. 28, 2000, pp. 1772–1776.
Crook, T.H., et al. "Effects of Phosphatidylserine in Age-Associated Memory Impairment." *Neurology,* Vol. 41, 1991, pp. 644–649.
Crook, T., et al. "Effects of phosphatidylserine in Alzheimer's disease." *Psychopharmacolgy Bulletin.* Vol. 28, 1992, pp. 61–66.
Cross, L.D. "Carpal Tunnel Syndrome, Epidemic of the 90s." *Health Naturally.* April/May, 1998, pp. 34–37.
"Cysteine." http://en.wikipedia.org/wiki/
Daly, J.M., et al. 1992. Enteral nutrition with supplemental arginine, RNA, and omega-3 fatty acids in patients after operation:immunologic, metabolic, and clinical outcome. *Surgery* 112:56-67.
Damrau, F. "Benign prostatic hypertrophy: amino acid therapy for symptomatic relief." *Journal American Geriatric Society,* Vol. 10, 1962, pp. 426–430.
Davies, Stephen and Alan Stewart. *Nutritional Medicine* (Vol 1). New York: Avon Books, 1987.
Davis, Joel. *Endorphins, New Wave of Brain Chemistry.* New York, NY: The Dial Press, 1984.

Dean, Ward and Jim English. *Vitamin Research News 2000 Anthology.* Carson City, NV: Vitamin Research Products, Inc., April, p. 2.

Debant, J.P. and L.A. Cynober. "Amino acids with anabolic properties." *Current Opinions in Clinical Nutrition and Metabolic Care.* Vol. 1, 1998, pp. 263–272.

Devlin, T. M. *Textbook of Biochemistry.* New York, NY: Wiley, 1982.

Dey, Lucy, Anoja S. Attele, and Chun-Su Yan. "Alternative Therapies for Type 2 Diabetes." *Alternative Medicine Review.* Vol. 7, No. 1, 2002, pp. 45–58.

Dodson W., Sach D., Krauss S., et al. "Alterations of serum and urinary carnitine profiles in cancer patients. Hypothesis of possible significance." *Journal American College of Nutrition.* Vol. 8, 1989, pp. 133–142.

Donati, L. et al. "Nutritional and clinical efficacy of ornithine alpha-ketoglutarate in severe burn patients." *Clinical Nutrition.* Vol. 18, 1999, pp. 307–311.

Doolittle TH, S.L. Hauser, et al. "Antispasticity Effect of Threonine in Multiple Sclerosis." *Archives of Neurology.* Vol.49, September 1992, pp. 923–926.

Ellis, John M. and Jean Pamplin. *Vitamin B6 Therapy.* Garden City Park: Avery Publishing, 199, pp. 1–45, 101–150.

Feinblatt, H.M. and J. C. Gant. "Pallative treatment for benign prostatic hypertrophy. Value of glycine-alanine-glutamic acids combination." *Journal Maine Medical Association.* Vol. 49, 1958, pp. 99–101, 124.

Ferrari E., D. Casarotti, M Muzzoni, et al. "Age related changes of the adrenal secretory pattern: possible role in pathological brain aging." *Brain Research Review.* November 2001, Vol. 37. No. 1–3, pp. 294–300.

Finkelstein J.D., J.J. Martin, and B.J. Harris. "Methionine metabolism in mammals. The methionine-sparing effect of cystine." *Journal of Nutritional Biochemistry.* Aug. 25,1988, Vol. 263, No. 24, pp. 11750–11754.

Flodin, N.W. "The metabolic roles, pharmacology, and toxicology of lysine." *Journal American College Nutrition,* Vol. 16, 1997, pp. 7–21.

Formica, P.E. "The housewife syndrome: treatment with the potassium and magnesium salts of aspartic acid." *Current Therapy Research.* Vol. 4, 1962, p. 98.

"Four Prespectives on Carpal Tunnel Syndrome," Your Health. Asheville, NC: *International Academy of Nutrition and Preventive Medicine.* Vol. XIII No. III, 1992.

Fox, Arnold and Barry Fox. *DLPA To End Chronic Pain and Depression.* New York: Long Shadow Books, 1985.

Fox, Barry. "C-Reactive Protein (CRP) – A New Blood Marker for Coronary Vascular Disease." *Journal of the American Nutraceutical Association,* Vol. 8, No. 1, pp. 43–45.

Fukuda, N., T. Hidaka T. Toda, M. Sugano. "Altered hepatic metabolism of free fatty acid in rats fed a threonine-imbalanced diet." *Journal of Nutrition Science Vitaminol* (Tokyo). Oct1990, Vol. 36, No. 5, pp. 467–474.

Furst, P. "Dietary L-Lysine supplementation, a promising nutritional tool in the prophylaxis and treatment of osteoporosis." *Nutrition.* Vol. 9., No. 1 1993, pp. 71–72.

Gaby, Alan. *B6, The Natural Healer.* New Canaan, CT: Keats Publishing, 1984.

Gaby, Alan R. "L-arginine for interstitital cystitis." *Townsend Letter for Doctors and Patients,* April 2001, #192, p. 32.

Gaby, Alan R. "L-arginine for dementia." *Townsend Letter for Doctors and Patients,* July 2002, #228, p. 24.

Gaby, Alan R. *Magnesium.* New Canaan, CT: Keats Publishing, 1994.

Gaby, Alan R. *Nutritional Medicine.* Fritz Perlberg Publishing, Concord, NH, 2011, pp. 587–594, 950–955.

Gaster, Barak. "S-adenosylmethionine (SAMe) for the Treatment of Depression." *Alternative Medicine* Alert. December 1999, p. 133–135.

Gelenberg, A. J. et al. "Tyrosine treatment of depression." *American Journal of Psychiatry.* Vol. 137, 1980, p. 622.

Gerber, James. *Handbook of Therapeutic and Preventative Nutrition.* Gaithersburg, MD: Aspen, 1993, pp. 244–245.

Gershon, Michael D. *The Second Brain.* New York: HarperCollins Publishers, 1998.

Ginkgo biloba leaf extract. Newton, MA: Lippincott Williams & Wilkins. 2000:359–366.

Gitlin, Michael. *The Psychotherapist's Guide to Psychopharmacology.* New York: The Free Press, 1990.

Goepp, Julius. "The overlooked compound that saves lives." *Life Extension magazine,* May 2010, pp. 64–74.

Goldberg, Burton, et al. *Alternative Medicine Guide to Heart Disease.* Tiburon, CA: Future Medicine Publishing. 1998.

Granat, Q. and J. DiMichele. "Phosphatidylserine in Elderly Patients. An Open Trial." *Clinical Trials Journal.* Vol. 24, 1987, pp. 99–103.

Grant W.B. An ecologic study of dietary and solar UV-B links to breast carcinoma mortality rates. *Cancer.* 2002a;94:272-81

Griffith, R., D.De long, and C. Kagan. *Dermatologia.* No. 156, pp. 257–267, 1978.

Griffith, R.S., et al. "Success of L-Lysine therapy in frequently recurrent herpes simplex infection; Treatment and prophylaxis." *Dermatologia.* Vol. 175, No. 4, pp. 183–190.

Harrison, Tinsley R., Thorn, George W. (ed), et al. *Harrison's Principles of Internal Medicine.* 8th Ed. New York: McGraw-Hill Book Co, 1977.

Heys, S.D., et al. "Dietary suppplementation with L-arginine: modulation of tumour-infiltrating lymphocytes in patients with colorectal cancer." *British Journal of Surgery, 1997* Vol. 84: pp.238–41.

Hicks, J.T. "Treatment of fatigue in general practice: a double-blind study." *Clinical Medicine.* January 1964, p. 85.

Hoffer, Abram and Morton Walker. *Orthomolecular Nutrition.* New Canaan, CT: Keats Publishing, 1978.

Hosking G.P., N.P. Cavanaugh, D.P. Symth, et al. "Oral treatment of Carnitine Mypopathy." *Lancet.* Vol. 16, 1977, p. 853.

Huxtable, R. J. and H. Pasantes-Morales. *Taurine in Nutrition and Neurology.* New York, NY: Plenium Press, 1981.

Huxtable, R. J. "Physiological Actions of Taurine." *Physiology Review.* Vol. 72, pp. 101–103.

Harper, H. A. *Review of Physiological Chemistry.* 12th Ed. Los Altos, CA: Lange Medical Publications, 1969, p. 29.

Hellhammer, J., E. Fries, C. Buss, et al. "Effects of soy lecithin phosphatidic acid and phosphatidylserine complex (PAS) on the endocrine and psychological responses to mental stress." *Stress.* June 2004, Vol .7, No. 1, pp. 119–126.

Herbs & Supplements: Taurine. Swedish Hospital. "Sources of Taurine." http://www.swedish.org/110983.cfm

"Herbs at a Glance: Ginkgo." *NCCAM (National Center for Complementary and Alternative Medicine) Publication* No. D290 September 2005, http://nccam.nih.gov/health/ginkgo/#cautions.

Holick, M.F. Vitamin D: importance in the prevention of cancers, type 1 diabetes, heart disease, and osteoporosis. *Am J Clin Nutr.* 2004;79:362-71.

Houdijk, A.P., E.R. Rijnsburger, J. Jansen, et al. "Randomized trial of glutamine-enriched enteral nutrition on infectious morbidity in patients with multiple trauma." *Lancet.* Vol. 352, 1998; pp. 772–776.

Houston, Mark C. "The Biochemistry, Pathogenesis, and Clinical Aspects of New, Extended, and Emerging Cardiovascular Risk Factors and Inflammatory Markers for Vascular Disease." Tenth International Symposium on Functional Medicine, Nutritional Biochemistry of the Cardiovascular System Pre-Course. May 22, 2003, Tucson, AZ

Houston, Mark C. "The Role of Vascular Biology, Nutrition and Nutraceuticals in the Prevention and Treatment of Hypertension." The Tenth International Symposium on Functional Medicine, Nutritional Biochemistry of the Cardiovascular System. May 22–25, 2003, Tucson, AZ

Houston, Mark C. and Ralph Hawkins. *Hypertension Handbook for Clinicians and Students.* Birmingham, AL: ANA Publishing, 2005, p. 49.

Hurot, J. M., et al. "Effects of L-carnitine supplementation in maintenance hemodialysis patients: a systemic review." *Journal American Society Nephrology.* Vol. 13, pp. 708–714.

Husband, Alan J. "Red Clover Isoflavone Supplements: Safety and Pharmacokinetics." *Journal of the British Menopause Society,* Supplement S1, 2001, p.4.

Isaacs H., J. Heffron, M. Badenhorst, et al. "Weakness Associated with the Pathological Presence of Lipid in Skeletal Muscle: A Detailed Study of a Patient with Carnitine Deficiency." *Journal of Neurology, Neurosurgery and Psychiatry.* Vol. 39, 1976, pp. 1114–1123.

"Is Dietary Cholesterol Really Public Enemy #1?" *Women's Health Connection*. Vol. VI, Issue I, 1999.

"Isoflavones in the Management of Menopause." *The Journal of the British Menopause Society*. Vol. 7, Supp. 1, 2001, Proceedings Supplement from an Educational Meeting.

James, Susan Donaldson. "Anxiety in Your Head Could Come From Your Gut." *ABC News' Good Morning America*. Sept. 12, 2013.

Jeevanadam, M. and S.R. Peterson. "Substrate fuel kinetics in enterally fed trauma patients supplemented with ornithine alpha-ketoglutarate." *Journal of Experimental Biology and Medicine*. Vol. 18, 1999, pp. 209–217.

Kagan, C. "Lysine Therapy for Herpes Simplex." *The Lancet*. Vol. 1, No. 37, 1974.

Keast, D., Arstein, D., et al. "Depression of plasma glutamine concentration after exercise stress and its possible influence on the immune system." *Medical Journal of Australia*. Vol. 162, 1995, pp. 15-18.

Kelly, Gregory S. "Sports Nutrition: A review of selected nutritional supplements for bodybuilders and strength athletes." *Medicine in Review*, Vol. 2, 1997, pp. 184–201.

Kelly, Gregory S. "Insulin Resistance: Lifestyle and Nutritional Interventions." *Alternative Medicine Review*. Vol. 5, No. 2, 2000, pp. 109–132.

Kidd, Parris M. "Glutathione: Systemic protectant against oxidative and free radical damage." *Alternative Medicine Review*. Vol. 2, No. 3, 1997, pp. 155–176.

Klatz, Ronald and Carol Kahn. *Grow Young with HGH*. New York: HarperCollins, 1998.

Klimberg, V.S. and J.L. McClellan. "Glutamine, cancer, and its therapy." *American Journal of Surgery*. Vol. 172, 1996, pp. 418–424.

Klotter, Jule. "Arginine and heart disease." *Townsend Letter for Doctors and Patients*. August–September 2002, p. 76–79.

Kotulak, Ronald. *Inside the Brain*. Kansas City: Andrew and McMeel, 1996.

Korting, G.E., et al. "A randomized double-bind trial of oral L-arginine for treatment of interstitial cystitis. *Journal of Urology*, 1999, Vol. 161, pp. 558–565.

Kruse, C.A. "Treatment of fatigue with aspartic acid salts." *Northwest Medicine.* June 1961, p. 257.

Kroger, H., A. Hauschild, and M. Ohme, et al. "Nicotinamide and methionine reduce the liver toxic effects of methotrexate." *General Pharmacology.* Vol. 33, 1999, pp. 203–206.

Kudsk, K.A., M.A. Croce, T.C. Fabian, et al. "Enteral versus parenteral feeding." *Annuals of Surgery.* Vol.215, 1992, pp. 503–511.

Kwyer, Thomas. "Glutathione depleting agents." http://www.fda.gov/ohrms/dockets/ac/00/slides/3652s1_05/sld028.htm

Kwyer, Thomas. "Glutathione: L-glutamylcysteinylgylcine" http://www.fda.gov/ohrms/dockets/ac/00/slides/3652s1_05/sld003.htm

Lacour, B., S. DiGiulio, J. Chanard, et al. "Carnitine improves lipid anomalies in hemodialysis patient." *Lancet.* October 11, 1978, pp. 763–764.

Le Boucher, et al. "Modulation of immune response with ornithine A-ketoglutarate in burn injury: an arginine or glutamine dependency?" *Nutrition.* Vol. 15, 1999, pp. 773–777.

Lee, A.L., W.O. Ogle, R.M. Sapolsky. "Stress and depression: possible links to neuron death in the hippocampus." *Bipolar Disorders,* April 2002, Vol. 4, No. 2, pp. 117–128.

Lee, John R. with Virginia Hopkins. *What Your Doctor May Not Tell You About Menopause.* New York: Warner Books, 1996, pp. 64, 285, 300–305.

Leibovitz, Brian. *Carnitine, The Vitamin Bt Phenomenon.* NY: New York: Dell Publishing, 1984.

Lemon, Peter. "Is increased dietary protein necessary or beneficial for individuals with a physically active livestyle?" *Nutrition Review.* Vol. 54, 1996, S169–175.

Li, J.B., Jefferson, L.S. *Biochemical Biophysical Acta.* 1978, pp. 351–359.

Lieber, C. S. and L. Packer. "S-Adenosylmethionine: molecular, biological, and clinical aspects–an introduction." *American Journal of Clinical Nutrition.* November 1, 2002; Vol. 76 No. 5, pp 1148–1150.

Liniger, S. (Ed.). *The Natural Pharmacy.* Rocklin, CA: Prima Health Publishing, 1998.

Lomaestro, B.M. "Glutathione in health and disease: pharmacotherapeutic issues." *Annuals of Pharmacotherapy.* December 1995, Vol. 12, pp. 1263–1273.

Lotan, R., et al. "The Effect of Lysine and Threonine Supplementation on the Immune Response of Growing Rats Fed Wheat Gluten Diets." *Nutrition Reports International.* 1980, Vol. 22 No. 3, pp. 313–318.

Maes, M., et al. "Serum Levels of Excitatory Amino Acids, Serine, Glycine, Histidine, Threonine, Taurine, Alanine and Arginine in Treatment-resistant Depression: Modulation by Treatment with Antidepressants and Prediction of Clinical Responsivity." *Acta psychiatrica Scandinavica.* April 1998, Vol. 97 No. 4, pp. 302–308.

MacKay, Douglas and Alan L. Miller. "Nutritional Support for Wound Healing." *Alternative Medicine Review.* Vol. 8, No. 14, pp. 359–377.

MacLennan, P.A., Smith, K., et al. "Inhibition of protein breakdown by glutamine in perfused rat skeletal muscle." *FEBS (Federation of Biochemical Societies) Letter,* Vol. 257, 1988, pp. 133–136.

Maher, Timothy J. "L-Arginine Continuing Education Module." *New Hope Institute.* February 2000, pp. 2–7.

Marchetti, G., et al. "Use of N-acetylcysteine in the management of coronary artery diseases." *Cardiolgia.* Vol. 44, No.7, July 1999, pp. 633–637.

Mayo Clinic Staff. "Anti-aging therapies: too good to be true?" www.mayoclinic.com *Senior Health Center,* HQ00233, May, 11, 2005.

Maxwell, Andrew J. and Cooke, John P. "Cardiovascular effects of L-arginine." *Current Opinion in Nephrology and Hypertension.* Vol. 7, January 1998, pp. 63–70.

Mendell, J.R., R.C. Griggs, R.T. Moxley III, et al. "Clinical investigation in Duchenne muscular dystrophy: IV. Double blind controlled trial of leucine." *Muscle Nerve.* Vol. 7, 1984, pp. 535, 541.

Mervyn, Len. *Minerals and Your Health.* New Canaan, CT: Keats Publishing, 1980, pp.36–40, 79–81.

"Methionine." Yalenewhavenhealth.org/library/health/guide/en-us/cam/topic.asp havoid=ln2884088.

Milne, Robert, et. al. *Definitive Guide to Headaches.* Tiburon, CA: Future Medicine Publishing, 1998.

Miller, Alan L. "Therapeutic Consideration of L-Glutamine: A Review of Literature." *Alternative Medicine Review.* Vol. 4, 1999; pp. 239–248.

Miller, Philip L. and Life Extension Foundation with Monica Reinagel. *The Life Extension Revolution.* New York: A Lynn Sonberg Book, Bantam Books, pp. 55–73.

Mills, Dixie. "Menopause—Ending the Confusion." http://www.womentowomen.com/menopause/index.asp

Moore, F.A., E.E. Moore, T.N. Jones, et al. TEN versus TPN following major abdominal trauma and reduced septic morbidity." *Journal of Trauma.* Vol. 29, 1989; pp. 916–923.

Moore, Thomas. *Prescription for Disaster.* New York: Simon & Schuster, 1998.

Morlion, B.J., P. Stehle, P. Wachter, et al. "Total parenteral nutrition with glutamine dipeptide after major abdominal surgery." *Annuals of Surgery.* Vol. 227, 1998, pp. 302–308.

Mowrey, Daniel. *Herbal Tonic Therapies.* New Canaan, CT: Keats Publishing, 1993.

Moyers, Bill. *Healing and the Mind.* New York: Doubleday, 1993.

Murray, M.T. and J. Pizzorno. *Encyclopedia of Natural Medicine.* 2nd Ed. Rocklin, CA: Prima Publishing, 1998.

Murray, Michael T. *The Healing Power of Herbs.* Rocklin, CA: Prima Publishing, 1995, p. 208.

Murray, Michael T. "The Many Benefits of Carnitine." *The American Journal of Natural Medicine.* March, 1966, pp. 6–13.

Nachtigall, Lila E. "Isoflavones in the management of menopause. *Journal of the British Menopause Society.* Supplement S1, 2001, pp. 8–11.

NCI Fact Sheet: Tea and Cancer Prevention. National Cancer Institute, U.S. National Institutes of Health Fact Sheet. 12/6/2002.

NCI Fact Sheet: Antioxidants and Cancer Prevention: Questions and Answers. National Cancer Institute, U.S. National Institutes of Health Fact Sheet. 7/2/2004.

Neu, J, V. De Marco, and N. Li. "Glutamine: clinical applications and mechanisms of action. *Current Opinions in Clinical Nutrition and Metabolic Care.* Vol. 5, 2002, pp. 69–72.

Neuborne, Ellen. "Workers in pain; employers up in arms." *USA Today,* January 9, 1997, Section B, p. 1–2.

Newbold, H.L. *Mega-Nutrients for Your Nerves.* New York: Peter Wyden, Publishing, 1975.

Newsholme, E.A. "Biochemical mechanisms to explain immunosuppression in well-trained and overtrained athletes." *International Journal of Sports Medicine,* Vol. 15, 1994; pp. S142–S147.

Nordiac Naturals. *Essential Fatty Acids: Omega-3 / Omega-6 Clinical Handbook.* Watsonville, CA. Monograph 2005.

Nutrition Data. "999 Foods Highest in Alanine." http://www.nutritiondata.com/foods--00009100000000000000.html Sept. 28, 2005.

Nutrition Data. "999 Foods Highest in Arginine." http://www.nutritiondata.com/foods-00009500000000000000.html

Nutrition Data. "999 Foods Highest in Aspartic Acid." http://www.nutritiondata.com/foods--00009100000000000000.html Sept. 28, 2005.

Nutrition Data. "999 Foods Highest in Cystine." http://www.nutritiondata.com/foods--00008500000000000000.html Sept. 27, 2005.

Nutrition Data. "999 Foods Highest in Glycine." http://www.nutritiondata.com/foods--00009400000000000000.html Sept. 27, 2005.

Nutrition Data. "999 Foods Highest in Glutamic Acid." http://www.nutritiondata.com/foods--00009300000000000000.html Sept. 27, 2005.

Nutrition Data. "999 Foods Highest in Glycine." http://www.nutritiondata.com/foods-00009400000000000000.html Nov. 14, 2005.

Nutrition Data. "999 Foods Highest in Histidine." http://www.nutritiondata.com/foods--00009000000000000000.html Sept. 27, 2005.

Nutrition Data. "999 Foods Highest in Isoleucine." http://www.nutritiondata.com/foods-00008100000000000000-1.html Nov. 3, 2005.

Nutrition Data. "999 Foods Highest in Lysine." http://www.nutritiondata.com/foods--00008900000000000000.html Sept. 28, 2005.
Nutrition Data. "999 Foods Highest in Methionine." http://www.nutritiondata.com/foods-000084000000000000000-7.html November 14, 2005.
Nutrition Data. "999 Foods Highest in Phenylalanine." http://www.nutritiondata.com/foods-000086000000000000000-2.html November 14, 2005.
Nutrition Data. "999 Foods Highest in Proline." http://www.nutritiondata.com/foods-000095000000000000000-20.html November 14, 2005
Nutrition Data. "999 Foods Highest in Serine." http://www.nutritiondata.com/foods--00009600000000000000.html Sept. 28, 2005.
Nutrition Data. "999 Foods Highest in Threonine." http://www.nutritiondata.com/foods-000080000000000000000-7.html Nov. 14, 2005.
Nutrition Data. "999 Foods Highest in Valine." http://www.nutritiondata.com/foods-000088000000000000000-9.html November 3, 2005.
Okumoto, S., et al. "Detection of glutamate release from neurons by genetically encoded surface-displayed FRET nanosensors." Proceedings of the *National Academy of Sciences*. U.S.A, June 14, 2005. Vol.102, No. 24, pp. 8740–8745.
Parry-Billings, M., et al. "A communicational link between skeletal muscle, brain, and cells of the immune system." *International Journal of Sports Medicine*. Vol. 11, 1990, pp. S122–S123.
Pasantes-Morales, Herminia et al. eds. *Taurine: Functional Neurochemistry, Physiology, and Cardiology.* New York: Wiley-Liss, 1990.
Patton, Dominique. "Omega-3s could lower risk of dry eye syndrome." Nutra Ingredients-USA Newsletter 10/18/2005 http://nutraingredients-usa.com/news/ng.asp?n=63288-omega-eye-fish
Perry, H.E. and M.W. Shannon. "Efficacy of oral versus N-acetylcysteine in acetaminophen overdose; results of an open label, clinical trial." *Journal of Pediatrics*. Vol. 132, No. 1, January 1998, pp. 149–152.

Pert, Candace B. *Molecules of Emotion.* New York: Scribner Publishing, 1997.

Pfeiffer, Carl. *Mental and Elemental Nutrition.* New Canaan, CT: Keats Publishing, 1975.

Pfeiffer, Carl. *Nutrition and Mental Illness.* Rochester, VT: Healing Arts Press, 1987.

Pizzuli, L., et al. "N-acetylcysteine attenuates nitroglycerin tolerance in patients with angia pectoris and normal left ventricular function." *American Journal of Cardiology.* Vol. 79, 1997, pp. 28–33.

Poortmans, J.R., and Hans Howard H. Metabolic Adaptation to Prolonged Physical Exercise. Basel, Switzerland: Birkhauseer Verlag, 1975, p. 212–228.

Prusinev, Stanley. *The Enzymes of Glutamine Metabolism.* New York, NY: Academic Press, 1973.

Raber, J. "Detrimental effects of chronic hypothalamic-pituitary-adrenal axis activation. From obesity to memory deficits." *Molecular Biology,* August 1998, Vol. 18. No. 1, pp. 1–22.

Rapp, Doris. *Is This Your Child's World?* New York: Bantam Books, 1996.

Redfern, Robert. *Pain Relief, Inflammation Relief and Clear Arteries! The 2nd Gift from Silkworms is Serrapeptase.* UK, Cheshire, CW8 1NL: Naturally Healthy Publications, 2004, pp. 27, 55, 152.

Reiter, R.J., J.R. Calvo, M. Karbownik, et al. "Melatonin and its relation to the immune system and inflammation." *Alternative Medicine Rewiew.* Vol. 6, No. 3, 2001, pp. 334.

Reynolds, T.M. "The future of nutrition and wound healing." *Journal of Tissue Viability.* Vol. 11 No. 1, 2001, pp. 5–13.

"Riboflavin Zaps Migraines." *Vitamin Retailer.* May, 1998, pp. 53–54.

Roberts, Molly M. and Richard S. Lord. *Ion Handbook, Clinical Reference Manual for the ION Profile.* Norcross, GA: Metametrix Clinical Laboratory, 2005.

Roe, D.A. *Drug–Induced Nutritional Deficiencies.* Westport CT: AVI Publishing Co.,1976.

Rogers, L.L. "Glutamine in the Treatment of Alcoholism." *Quarterly Journal of Studies on Alcohol.* Vol. 18, No. 4., 1957, pp. 581–587.

Rogers, L.L. and R.B. Pelton. "Effect of Glutamine on IQ Scores of Mentally Deficient Children." *Texas Reports on Biology and Medicine.* Vol. 15, No. 1, 1957, pp. 84–90.

Rogers, Sherry A. *How to Cure Diabetes!* Sarasota, FL: Sand Key Co., Inc., 2013 pp. 104–140, 344.

Rogers, Sherry A. *Tired or Toxic?* Syracuse, NY: Prestige Publishing, 1990.

Rogers, Sherry A. *Wellness Against All Odds.* Syracuse, NY: Prestige Publishing, 1994.

Rogers, Sherry A. *Pain Free in 6 Weeks.* Sarasota, FL: Sand Key Co., Inc., 2001.

Rosisk, Edward R. "Cortisol, Stress and Health." *Life Extension.* December 2005, pp. 40–48.

Roumen, R.M., J.A. van der Vliet, R.A.Wevers, R.J. Goris. "Intestinal permeability is increased after major vascular surgery." *Journal of Vascular Surgery.* Vol. 17, 1993, pp. 734–737.

Roumen, R.M., T. Hendriks, R.A. Wevers, J.A. Goris. "Intestinal permeability after severe trauma and hemorrhagic shock is increased without relation to septic complications." *Archives of Surgery.* Vol. 128,1993, pp. 453–457.

Rowbottom, D.G., D. Keast, A.R. Morton. "The emerging role of glutamine as an indicator of exercise stress and overtraining." *Sports Medicine,* Vol. 21, 1996, pp. 80–97.

Sahley, Billie J. *The Anxiety Epidemic.* San Antonio, Texas: Pain & Stress Publications,® 2007.

Sahley, Billie J. and Katherine M. Birkner. *Break Your Prescribed Addiction.* San Antonio, TX: Pain & Stress Publications,® 2004.

Sahley, Billie J. *Stop A.D.D. Naturally.* San Antonio, TX: Pain & Stress Publications®, 2010.

Sahley, Billie J. *GABA, The Anxiety Amino Acid.* San Antonio, TX: Pain & Stress Publications®, 2005.

Segala, Melanie, Ed. *Disease Prevention and Treatment.* 4th Ed. Hollywood, FL: Life Extension Media., 2003, pp. 63, 126–127.

Shabert, Judy and Nancy Ehrlich. *The Ultimate Nutrient, Glutamine.* Garden City Park, NY: Avery Publishing, 1994.

Shaw, D.L. et al. "Management of fatigue: a physiological approach." *American Journal Medical Science.* 1962, pp. 243, 758.

Shaw, G. M. E. M. Velie, and D. M. Schaffer. "Is dietary intake of methionine associated with a reduction in risk for neural tube defect associated with pregnancies? *Teratology.* Vol. 56, pp. 295–259.

Sinatra, Stephen T. *The Sinatra Solution Metabolic Cardiology.* Laguna Beach, CA: Basic Health Publications, 2008, pp. 101–143.

Singer, P., et al. "Nutritional aspects of the Acquired Immunodeficiency Syndrome." *American Journal of Gastroenterology,* Vol. 87, 1992, pp. 265–273.

Singh, R., et al. 2000. Arginase activity in human breast cancer cell lines: NT-Hydroxy-L-arginine selectively inhibits cell proliferation and induces apoptosis in MDA-MB-468 cells. *Cancer Res.* 60:3305-12.

Smith, Robert. "Chronic Headaches in Family Practice." *Journal of the American Board of Family Practice.* Vol. 6, Nov/Dec, 1992, pp. 589–599.

Smithstein, M.J., et al. "Efficacy of oral N-acetylcysteine in the treatment of acetaminophen overdose." Analysis of the national multicenter study (1976 to 1985). *New England Journal of Medicine.* Vol. 319, No. 24, Dec. 15, 1988, pp. 1557–1562.

Souba, W.W. *Glutamine: physiology, biochemistry, and nutrition in critical illness.* Austin, TX: R.G. Landes Co., 1992.

Souba, W.W. "The gut as a nitrogen-processing organ in the metabolic response to critical illness." *Nutrition Support Services.* Vol., 1988, pp. 15–22.

Souba, Wiley W., et al. "Glutamine Metabolism by the Intestinal Tract." *Journal of Parenteral and Enteral Nutrition.* Vol. 9., No. 5 p. 608.

Smythies, J.R. and J.H. Halsey. "Treatment of Parkinson's disease with l-methionine." *Southern Medical Journal.* Vol. 77, 1984, p. 1577.

Taurine, A Monograph. *Alternative Medicine Review.* Vol. 6, No. 1, 2001, pp. 78–82.

Thomassen, A., et al. "Anti-ischemic and metabolic effects of glutaminate during pacing in patients with stable angina pectoris secondary to either coronary heart disease or syndrome X." *American Journal of Cardiology*. Vol. 125, 1991, pp. 2907–2915.

Thompsen J.H., A.L. Shug, V.U. Yap, et al: "Improved pacing tolerance of the ischemic human myocardium after administration of carnitine." *American Journal of Cardiology*. Vol. 43, 1979, pp. 300–305.

Thomson, J. et al. "The treatment of depression in general practice: a comparison of L-tryptophan, amitriptyline and combination with placebo." *Psychological Medicine.* December 1982, p. 741

Tischler, M. et al. *Journal Biological Chemistry.* Vol. 4, pp. 1613–1621.

Uden, S., D. Bilton, L. Nathan, et al. "Antioxidant therapy for recurrent pancreatitis: placebo-controlled trial." *Alimentary Pharmacology & Therapeutics*, Vol. 4, 1990, pp. 357–371.

Vale, J. A., T.J. Meredith, and R. Goulding. "Treatment of acetaminophen poisoning. The use of oral methionine." *Archives of Internal Medicine.* Vol. 141, 1981, pp. 141.

Vannice, Gretchen and Jill Kelly. "Mood Disorders and Omega-3 Fatty Acids." Watsonville, CA: Nordic Naturals, 2004, pp. 1–5.

Varanasi, R.V. and J.R. Saltzma. "Ornithine oxoglutarate therapy improves nutrition status." *Nutrition Review.* Vol. 53, 1996, pp. 96–97.

Vasdev, S., M. Whalen, et al. "Ethanol-and Threonine-induced Hypertension in Rats: A Common Mechanism." *Canadian Journal of Cardiology.* Vol. 11, No. 9, October 1995, pp. 807–815.

Vinnars, E., J. Bergstrom, and P. Furst. "Influence of the postoperative state on the intracellular free amino acids in human muscle tissue." *Annuals of Surgery.* Vol. 182, 1975, pp. 665–671.

Vuzelov, E., et al. "Plasma levels of branched chain amino acids in patients on regular dialysis before and after including a high-protein supplement in their diet."

Folic Medicine. Vol. 41, 1999, pp. 19–22.

Walsh, N.P., A.K. Blannin, P.J. Robson, and M. Gleeson. "Glutamine, exercise and immune function. Links and possible mechanisms." *Sports Medicine.* Vol. 26, 1998, pp. 77–191.

Wein, Harrison. "Migraines not in the mind." The NIH Word on Health, June 2000, http://www.nih.gov/news/WordonHealth/jun2000/story02.htm

Werbach, Melvyn. *Nutritional Influences on Mental Illness.* Tarzana, CA: Third Line Press, 1987, pp. 73, 119, 138–139, 192–193, 200.

Wernerman, J., F. Hammarkvist, M. Rustom, and E. Vinnars. "Glutamine and ornithine-alpha-ketoglutarate but not branched-chain amino acids reduce the loss of muscle glutamine after surgical trauma." *Metabolism.* Vol. 38,1989, pp. S63–S66.

Whitaker, Julian. "Diabetes Treatment Review: How to Take Control." *Health and Healing Newsletter.* September, 1995, pp. 1–4.

Whitaker, Julian. *Reversing Diabetes.* New York: Warner Books, 1987.

White, A. et al. *Principles of Biochemistry.* 6th Ed. New York, NY: McGraw-Hill, 1978.

Williams, R.J. *Alcoholism: The Nutritional Approach.* Austin, TX: Univ. of Texas Press, 1958, pp. 88, 100.

Wilmore, D.W. "Catabolic illness: strategies for enhancing recovery." *New England Journal of Medicine.* Vol. 325,1991, pp. 695–702.

Wilmore, D.W. "Metabolic support of the gastrointestinal tract. Potential gut protection during intensive cytotoxic therapy." *Cancer.* Vol. 79, 1997, pp. 1794–1803.

"Zest for Life, RDA of amino acids." http://anyvitamins.com/amino-acids/rda-amino-acids.htm

Ziegler, T.R., R.J. Smith, S.T. O'Dwyer, et al. "Increased intestinal permeability associated with infection in burn patients." *Archives of Surgery.* Vol. 123, 1988, pp. 1313–1319.

Index

Symbols
5-HTP (5-Hydroxytryptophan) 45, 78, 113, 130, 134, 136, 197, 220, 244
25-hydroxyvitamin D [25 (OH)D] 174
% Daily Value 16

A
acetaldehyde 42
acetaminophen 44, 59
acetylcholine 41, 45, 113, 117, 147
Acetyl-L-Carnitine (ALC) 40–42
acne 40, 93, 187
A.D.D. 14–15, 17, 97, 218
addiction, drug 251
addiction, tobacco 255
addictive behavior 95–96
adenosine triphosphate (ATP) 12, 61
ADHD 97–98, 114, 218
adrenal cortex 116
adrenaline (epinephrine) 13, 16–17, 133, 239
Advil 51
affective disorder 137
aggression 76–77, 219–220, 244, 249
aging 41, 104–106, 144, 241
agoraphobia 203
AIDS 206
ALA 114
alanine 20–21, 25, 80, 230, 246
alcohol 66, 233, 235
alcohol cravings 54
alcoholism 84, 95
alcohol withdrawal 56
Aleve 51
allergens 100
allergic reaction 88
allergies 93, 100, 107, 135
allergies, food 51, 185, 187, 228
allergy 157, 173–174
alpha keratin 42
alpha-ketoglutarate (OKG) 48, 63
Alpha-Ketoglutaric (Alpha KG) 90
Alpha Linolenic Acids (ALA) 107, 114
Alpha Lipoic Acid 169
ALS 74, 236, 243
Alzheimer's 41, 44, 48, 67, 114, 117, 147, 249
amino acid 23
amino acid analysis 90, 227
amino acid, conditionally essential 48, 68
amino acid, essential 21, 58
amino acid metabolism 227
amino acid, nonessential 21, 25, 30, 36, 47, 55, 66–67, 79
amino acids product grades 257
amino acids, proteogenic 20–21
amino acid testing 227
ammonia 17, 31, 47, 49, 63, 113, 230–232, 240
amphetamine 60
amygdala 24, 45, 73, 218
amyotropic lateral sclerosis (ALS) Lou Gehrig's disease 48
Anaprox 51
androgens 93
anemia 233
aneurysms 160
anger 24, 219–220
angina 29, 37, 163
anti-aging 249
anti-anxiety 14
antibiotics 177
antibody 58, 239
anticonvulsant 39
antidepressant 14, 60, 65, 78, 125, 133, 213, 245
anti-inflammatory 51, 237
anti-manic 14
antioxidant 163, 239
antitoxin 43
anxiety 11, 15, 23, 45–47, 62, 65, 75, 87, 234, 236
anxiety-related messages 17
appetite 240
arginine 20–21, 26, 29, 30, 48, 53, 63, 80, 148, 171, 230, 232, 240, 246
Aricept 41
arrhythmias 37, 69–70, 87, 98
arteriosclerosis 69
arthritis 240
arthritis, rheumatoid 57
asparagine 20–21, 30–31
aspartic acid 20–21, 48, 231, 246
ASPCA 155
asthma 87, 90, 107, 233
atherosclerosis 27, 29, 38, 85, 161, 164, 232
ATP (adenosine triphosphate) 31, 167
auditory nerves 237
autism 249
autoimmune 240
axon 14
AZT 40

B
B6 (pyridoxine) 17, 31, 47, 60, 67, 82, 85, 90, 239
bad breath (halitosis) 207
barbiturate 60
basal ganglia 45
BCAAs (Branched Chain Amino Acids) 31–33, 40, 238, 245
behavioral therapy 196, 204
benign prostatic hypertrophy (BPH) 48
Berkson, Burton 168
beta-amyloid 117
Bifidobacterium 177
bile 242
biochemical individuality 23
biochemical medicine 227
bipolar 61, 137

bird flu 44
blood-brain-barrier 16–19,
   49, 75–77, 106,
   134, 234–235
blood sugar 140
bone loss 86
BPH (benign prostatic
   hypertrophy) 25
brain 11, 16, 18, 26, 32,
   41, 45, 47, 49, 53,
   56, 65, 67, 70, 80,
   112, 125, 129, 156,
   197
brain chemistry 125, 130
brain drain 125
brain hemorrhages 160
brain waves 72
Branched Chain Amino
   Acids (BCAAs) 25
Breggin, Peter 97
bronchitis 233
Bronson, Phyllis 61
burns 50

C
caffeine withdrawal 160
cancer 28–29, 39, 50, 107,
   168, 173–195, 236,
   250
Candida 177
carbamezepine (Tegretol
   and Epitol) 39
carbohydrate 12, 31
cardiovascular 28, 38, 40,
   59, 60, 141
carnitine 21, 35–40,
   59–60, 147, 231
carnitine deficiency 36
carpal tunnel syndrome
   84, 119–120
cataracts 233
catecholamine 13, 65, 240,
   245
CCK (cholecystokinin) 65,
   240
cellular energy 31
central nervous system
   (CNS) 45, 47,
   74, 76
cerebellum 24, 68
cerebral cortex 24, 68
chelator 233
chemical imbalance 133
chemical intolerances 82
chemicals 225
chemotherapy 39, 49–50,
   235
Chinese club moss 114
chlorine 236

cholecystokinin 65
choleocephtokinin 240
cholesterol 29, 37, 60,
   163–164, 231, 250
choline 113, 59, 112, 239
chondrotin sulfate (CS)
   199–201
chromium 12, 84
Chronic Emotional Fatigue
   (CEF) 121
chronic fatigue 82
Chronic Fatigue Syndrome
   (CFS) 88
Chronic Stress Syndrome
   (CSS) 107, 121
circadian rhythms 77, 217
cirrhosis 30, 32, 66, 168,
   164, 230, 251
citric acid 90
citrulline 63, 232
Clayton Foundation 54
cluster 157
cluster headache 159
CoEnzyme Q10 160, 163
cognitive 67–68, 115
cognitive impairment 147
cohosh, black 193
collagen 20, 56, 58, 59,
   66, 74, 233, 238,
   240–241
concentration 17, 114, 54,
   73, 114–116, 206,
   219, 235, 254
conditionally essential
   amino acid 48, 68
congestive heart failure
   (CHF) 37, 39,
   69–72, 241, 252
contraceptives 93
convulsions 56, 66
coronary artery disease
   29, 38
coronary heart disease
   (CHD) 162, 232
cortex 24, 45, 117
cortisol 105, 108
cortisone 64, 120
craving alcohol 95
craving for sugar 56
C-Reactive Protein (CRP)
   164
creatine 26, 59
Crohn's disease 206
curcumin 200
Cylert 224
cysteine 20–21, 236, 241,
   42–43, 60, 68, 232,
   235, 240, 246
cystic fibrosis 241–242,

cystine 21, 233–234, 246
cystine 42

D
deanol 59
delta waves 72
dementia 28, 147–148
dental problems 160
depression 11, 23, 25,
   31–32, 45, 57,
   61–63, 66, 74–79,
   88, 116, 124, 130,
   132, 134, 136,
   138, 147, 152,
   176, 182, 185,
   190–191, 196,
   198, 203, 206,
   211, 217, 219,
   232, 236–237,
   243–244, 251
detoxifier 47
DHA (docosahexenoic
   acid) 98, 107,
   114, 147, 200
DHEA 106, 228
diabetes 29, 37, 63, 140,
   84, 87, 138, 206,
   251
diabetic retinopathy 84
Diamond, W. John 250
digestion 109
diuretics 90
dizziness 32
DL-Phenylalanine
   (DLPA) 66,
   128–130
DNA 31, 56, 67, 103
dopa 240, 245
dopamine 17, 61, 64, 72,
   134, 196, 240, 245
Down's syndrome 206
D-Ribose 167
drug addiction 251
drug-resistant seizure 25

E
eczema 234
EGCG (polyphenols) 74
elastin 74
emotion 22–23
emphysema
EMS (eosinophilia-my-
   algia syndrome)
   78
Emu oil 172
encephalopathy 33
endogenous morphine
   129
endorphins 66, 129

endothelial cells 26
endurance 32
energy 32, 33, 56, 237–238, 251
enteric nervous system 179
enzymes 20, 42, 58, 104, 108, 146
EPA (eicosapentaenoic acid) 98, 107, 114, 200
epilepsy 31,48, 70, 236, 241–242, 252
epinephrine (adrenalin) 13, 59, 64, 65, 113, 134, 132, 147, 240, 244–245
Epstein Barr virus 230, 239
essential amino acid 58–59, 74–75
Essential Fatty Acids (EFAs) 107, 228
estrogen 107
Exelon 41
exercise 52
exercise endurance 231
exposure therapy 204
eye 71
eyestrain 160

F
fatigue 32, 82, 87–88, 91, 105, 120–124, 198, 211
fatigue, chronic 82
fatty acids 11, 147, 215, 228
fatty liver 30
fear 17, 23–24, 65, 124, 126
fever 32, 49
fibromyalgia 57, 82, 87–88, 131, 133
fibromyalgia 87
fight-or-flight response 65
fight-or-flight syndrome 45
flashbacks 211–212
flora 176–178
flu 44
flu, bird 44
focus 73
folic acid 67
Folkers, Karl 84
food allergy 157, 180, 188, 199, 228, 235
food sensitivities/allergies 180, 188

free radical 103, 104, 141, 236
frontal lobe 197

G
GABA (Gamma Amino Butyric Acid) 17, 20, 22–24, 45, 47, 53, 68, 70, 72, 73, 80, 95, 134, 136, 220, 234
Galantamind 117
gallbladder 71, 252
gallstones 71
Gelenberg, Alan 17, 79, 134
genes 10, 220
Gershon, Michael 179
gingivitis 206
ginkgo biloba 54, 114
glaucoma 160
glucocorticoid 51
glucosamine 199
glucose 16, 55
glucose tolerance factor 235
glutamic acid (glutamate) 20–21,47, 53, 66, 234–236
glutamine 17, 20–21, 24–25, 47, 49, 53, 54, 63, 80, 113, 132, 134, 147, 206, 220, 235, 239–240
glutathione 236, 43, 56, 59, 104, 235
glycine 17, 21, 25, 47, 56–57, 68, 70, 74, 80, 235–237, 243, 246
glycogen 55
glycoproteins 67
goiter 175
Golden, Gerald 223
gout 48
Greenblatt, James 203
green tea 72–74, 132, 134
grief 23, 151, 148
growth hormone 26, 51, 53, 63, 232, 239–240
gum disease 146
gut 204

H
hair loss 30
hawthorne 167
HDL (high density lipids) 37, 231

headache 32, 46, 133, 156–158
headache, avoidance 157
headache, cluster 159
headache, migraine 157
headache, occipital neuralgia 160
headache, sinus (congestion) 159, 162
headache, tension 158
head trauma 160
headache triggers 157
Healing Miracle 74
heart 74
heart disease 60, 84, 162, 159
heart failure 252
heavy metals 56, 59, 108, 239
hepatic encephalopathy
hepatitis 32
Hepatitis C 168, 252
herbicides 104
heroin 60
herpes 30, 58, 170, 238–239
herpes simplex 230
herpes zoster 58
hippocampus 24, 45, 53, 68, 113, 205, 218
histamine 237, 57, 60, 135, 88, 133, 236–239
histidine 20–21, 57, 80, 221, 208, 236, 246
HIV/AIDS 60
Hoffer 10
Holick, Michael 174
homeostasis 9
homocysteine 60–61, 84, 239
homocysteine, excess 60
hormonal imbalances 182
hormones 20, 31, 58, 93
Houston, Mark 27
human growth hormone (HGH) 63
huperzine 114
hydroxyproline 63
hyperactivity 15, 75, 82, 234, 236, 252
hypercholesterolemia 29
hypertension 29, 73, 87, 160-164, 253
hypoglycemia 30, 253
hypotension 240
hypothalamus 45, 57, 65, 68, 95

I

Ibuprofen 51
illness, chronic 250
Imipramine 224
immune 20
immune suppression 29
immune system 23, 49, 51, 54, 73, 105, 125, 144, 160, 163, 73–174, 176–177, 179, 185, 239–240
immunoglobulins 20, 185
immunomodulator 173
immunosuppressive 67
infantile spasms 31
infections 32, 238
infertility 175
inflammation 164, 168, 188, 191, 200, 245
inhibitory neurotransmitter 49, 53, 56
inositol 47
Inside the Brain 56
insomnia 75-77, 148, 182, 191, 216,–217, 240, 243-244, 253
insulin 12, 234
intermittent claudication 38
interstitial cystitis 28
intestinal permeability 235
iodine 175–177
iodine, deficiency 175
iron 36
iron deficiency 233
irritability 32
Irritable Bowel Syndrome (IBS) 87, 177, 179
isoleucine 20–21, 32, 76, 80, 237, 246
isoleucine deficiency 32

J

James, Susan D. 203

K

ketones 39
kidney disease 232
kidney stone 234
kidney stones 87–88
Klatz, Ronald 27, 105–106
Kotulak, Ronald 56, 205, 219
Krebs cycle (TCA cycle) 31, 90
Kulvinskas, Viktor 109
Kurlan, Roger 223

L

Lactobacillus 177
lead 56, 58–59, 236
leaky-gut syndrome
leaky gut syndrome (LGS) 51, 185
lecithin 59, 239
leg ulcers 253
leucine 20–21, 32–33, 76, 80, 246
leukemia 31
limbic system 17, 24, 45, 133, 205, 218
linoleic acid (LA) 107
liver 56
liver disease 164, 168, 253
liver regeneration 63
Lizza, E. F. 27
long-term memory 29
loss of control 46
L-T (L-Theanine) 134, 136
lung diseases 233
Luteolin (tetra-hydroxyflavone) 168
Luvox 78
lysine 20–21, 36, 53, 58, 80, 167, 171, 238, 247
lysine deficiency 59

M

macular degeneration 44, 83
Mag Link (magnesium chloride) 47, 87
magnesium 16, 69, 84, 90–91, 115, 159, 230
magnesium deficiency 87–88, 183
magnets 131, 161
Maher, Timothy 29
mania 61, 74, 137–138, 253
meditation 72, 134
mega dose 9–10
mega nutrient 9–10
melatonin 59, 77, 216–217
memories 11, 24, 212
memory 16, 28, 41, 53–54, 67, 79, 114, 116, 148, 235, 254
memory, long-term 29
meningitis 160
menopause 191
menstrual cramps 87
mental alertness 254
mercury 42, 107–108, 249
metals, heavy , 237
methionine 20–21, 36, 59, 68, 80, 200–201, 232, 239–241, 247
methotrexate 59
migraine 87, 157
mineral loss 146
mitochondria 12
mitral valve prolapse 87
mood 24, 54, 65, 133
mood stabilizer 244
mood swings 147, 160, 216
Motrin 51
Mowrey, Daniel 54
multiple sclerosis 74
muscle 32, 238–240
muscle spasms 46–47, 87, 121–122, 158, 201, 209, 215
muscle weakness 36
muscular dystrophy 38, 70, 235
myelin 57, 237

N

NAC (N-Acetyl Cysteine) 43, 104. 233
Naprosyn 51
National Institute of Health (NIH) 16
National Pet Loss Hotline 155
nausea and pregnancy 237
nephrosclerosis 29
neurohormone 76–77, 106, 216, 244
neurological defects 32
neuromodulator 242
neuromuscular pain 88
neuron 11–12, 19, 41, 68, 219
neuropeptide 22–24, 54
neurotoxicity 84
neurotransmitter 11–15, 16–17, 22–23, 28, 41, 43, 54, 57, 62, 66–68, 70, 75–77, 80, 112, 116, 129, 134, 146, 152, 197, 216–217, 220, 236
neurotransmitter imbalances 221
neurotransmitter, inhibitory 25, 134, 236
niacin 36, 244
niacinamide 47, 201

nicotinic acid 77
nightmares 211–212
nightshades 199
night sweats 191
NIH 50
nitric oxide (NO) 26–28
nitrogen 26
nitroglycerin 167
noise sensitivity 87
non-essential amino acid 42, 62
nonsteroidal anti-inflammatory medications (NSAIDs) 187, 201
noradrenaline (norepinephrine) 13
norepinephrine (noradrenaline) 13, 16, 45, 65–66, 79, 113, 133, 147, 240, 245
NSAIDS (Non Steroidal Anti-Inflammatory Drugs) 187, 201
nucleic acids 59

O

obsessive behavior 244
obsessive-compulsive disorder (OCD) 57, 195, 223
omega-3 fatty acids 29, 135, 200
opiate 22
Ornish, Dean 163
ornithine 28, 31, 48, 53, 63–64, 66
Ornithine alpha-ketoglutarate (OKG) 63
orotates 31
orthinine 28, 232, 240
orthomolecular therapy 9–10, 204
osteoarthritis 62, 198–201, 249
osteoporosis 58, 86

P

P5'P (Pyridoxal 5' Phosphate) 82, 85
pain 11, 45, 57, 65, 71, 75–76, 105, 128, 130, 244
pain, back and neck 87
pain, chronic 128, 133, 242, 250
Paleolithic diet 167

pancreas 18, 140
pancreatic enzyme insufficiency 109
pancreatin 109
pancreatitis 60
panic 15, 126, 179, 202
panic attack 46, 87, 202
panic disorder 202
Parkinson's 57, 60, 238, 244–245, 254
Pauling, Linus 16
PEA 66
pellagra 244
peptide 22–24,, 30, 64
perimenopause 191–192
periodontal disease 163, 206–207
peripheral vascular diseases 38
perodontis 206
peroxisomes 168
Pert, Candace 22–23, 45
pesticides 108
pet grief 155
pet loss 156
petrochemicals 236
pets 71
Pfeiffer, Carl 9
phenylalanine 13, 20–21, 64, 76, 80, 113, 147, 240, 247
Phenylketonurics (PKU) 63–64
Philpott, William 43
phobias 57, 217
phosphatidylserine (PS) 67, 108, 115
phospholipids 56, 67
PhytoBalance 193
pimples 93
pineal gland 68
pituitary gland 26, 240
PKU (phenylketonuria) 63–64
PMS (Premenstrual Syndrome) 84, 88, 207–208
pneumonia 52
pollens 225
pollution 104, 233
poor wound healing 30
postmenopausal 163
post synaptic receptor 14
Post Traumatic Stress Disorder (PTSD) 211
PoweRelief 172
pregnancy 84, 243
pregnenolone 116
Premenstrual Syndrome (PMS) 207–209

product info 257
proline 20–21, 48, 63, 66, 240–241, 247
prostaglandins 104
proteinase 20
proteins 11, 20
proteoglycans 199
Prozac 220
psoriasis 234
psychoactive 73
psychoneuroimmunology 23
psychosis 67
psychosomatic 124
psychotropic 61
PTSD (Post Traumatic Stress Disorder) 211
pumpkin seed oil 194
Pyridoxal 5' Phosphate (P5'P) 17, 80, 82, 85, 113
pyrimidine 31

Q
R

radiation 104, 233, 235, 254
Radomski 26
Rapp, Doris 224
renal failure 32, 254
stress injury (RSI) 84, 119
retina 71
retinal (eye) degeneration 241
retinitis pigmentosa 71
rheumatoid arthritis 237
Ritalin 97–98, 223
RNA 29
Roberts, Eugene 45
Rogers, Lorene 55
Rogers, Sherry 70, 224

S

saline 100
SAMe 200–201
SAMe (S-Adenosyl Methionine) 61
schizophrenia 30–31, 48, 60, 231, 244, 254
Seasonal Affective Disorder (SAD) 215
Seelig, Mildred 90
seizure 25, 31, 56, 66, 87, 242, 254
selenium 60, 169
sepsis 32–33, 50

serine 20–21, 59, 67, 74, 232, 247
serotonin 14, 24, 31, 34, 62, 72, 76, 78, 113, 130, 133–134, 147, 196–197, 219, 221
serotonin syndrome 62
serrapeptase 200
Serzone 220
Shabert, Judy 51
Shealy, Norman 106
Silymarin 169
sinus 157, 233
sinus headache 162
Sjogren's syndrome 44
sleep cycle 77
sleep disorders 77
smoking 162–164
SNRI (Serotonin Norepinephrine Reuptake Inhibitors) 62
spastic 56
SSRI (Selective Serotonin Reuptake Inhibitors) 61
stamina 91
steroids 34
stress 11, 14, 17, 23, 32, 34, 45, 49, 51, 65, 69, 71, 74, 79, 82, 116, 141, 144, 176, 179,182, 223–234, 237–238, 254–255
stress amino acid 86, 105, 116, 123, 133, 188, 245
stress, chronic 123, 188
stress hormone 105, 116
stress mineral 86
stroke 31, 60, 157, 160
substance abuse 212
sugar craving 17
sulfur amino acid 233, 239
Sumner, James B. 109
superhormones 116
surgery 32, 50–51, 64, 238, 255
synapse 14, 19, 65
synaptic cleft 14
Syndrome X 141
systemic infections (sepsis) 160

T

tardive dyskinesia 255
taurine 21, 241, 48, 60, 68, 70, 80, 144, 147, 240, 247
taurine deficiency 70–71
teenagers 218
Tegretol 39
temper 73
Temporomandibular Joint Dysfunction (TMJ) 159
tension 157
tension headache 158
tension, muscle 234
tension (muscle) contraction 157
testosterone 35, 106–107
thalamus 45
theanine 20–21, 72, 74, 247
theophylline
Theta brain waves 72
The Ultimate Nutrient Glutamine 51
threonine 20–21, 74, 242–243, 247
thymus gland 74
thyroid 245
tics 70, 222, 210, 223
tics, motor 222
tobacco 255
tobacco addiction 255
Tofranil 78
tooth enamel 74
Tourette's 70, 222, 224
tranquilizers 46
trauma 32, 49, 64, 211–213, 238
tremors 32, 62
trigger point 158, 161
triglycerides 37
trypsinogen 42
tryptophan 14, 20–21, 34, 112–113, 76–77, 144, 147, 243–245, 247
tryptophan pathway 75
turmeric 200
twitches 62, 223, 209
tyrosine 13, 17, 20–21, 76–77, 113, 132, 134, 144, 147, 244–245, 247
tyrosine 64

U

uncertainty 65
unipolar depression 76

urea 30, 240
urea cycle 240
uremia 38, 232

V

valine 20–21, 32–34, 76, 80, 244–245, 247
valine deficiency 32
valproic acid (Depakote) 39
vascular dementia 147
vegetarians 238–239
vertigo (dizziness) 34, 87
Viagra 27
violence 220
viral growth 58
Vitamin B6 43, 53, 59, 76, 83
Vitamin B12 239
Vitamin C 16, 36, 37, 42, 66, 90, 104, 236–237
Vitamin D 173
Vitamins B 16
Vitamins B6 36
Vitamins E 104
Voaden 71

W

wakefulness 72
waves, alpha 72, 132, 134
waves, beta 72
weight control 244, 255
weight lifting 238
Whitaker, Julian 141
Williams, Roger 53–54, 112–113
Wilmore, Douglas 51
withdrawal, caffeine 160
wound healing 63, 240

X

Xanax 46

Y

Z

zinc 68, 84, 240–241
Zoloft 220
Zorgniotti, A.W. 27

Other Books
From Pain & Stress Publications

Hurt All Over? Answers!

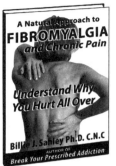

Get relief from pain, depression, and feelings of hopelessness using naturally.

The nutritional approach *offers hope and long-term relief* without the uncomfortable side effects of medications. A complete easy-to-follow program is outlined.

Begin to live again without pain. Get answers to help your healing process begin, and your constant pain diminish.

Control Anxiety and Stress Naturally

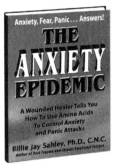

A wounded healer takes you through her own five-year battle with panic, fear, and phobias.

Learn how she healed herself with vital brain nutrients. Understand what causes feelings of anxiety and how to overcome it without drugs.

Learn how to use amino acids and control your anxiety.

Can't Live Without Your Meds? Addicted?

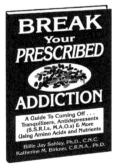

A step-by-step guide to coming off tranquilizers and antidepressants.

For every prescription drug, *there is a nutrient that does the exact same thing in the brain!*

Outlines specific amino acids and nutrients with suggested doses that support the brain during withdrawal.

Outlines a *safe withdrawal* and maintenance program.

Ritalin and Other Drugs are NOT the Answer to ADD & ADHD!

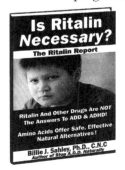

Amino Acids offer safe, effective natural alternatives to Ritalin and other drugs.

This booklet is a *must* for parents, educators and health care practitioners.

It details information not only about Ritalin, but other addictive medications used for children.

To Order Call 1-800-669-2256 or go to www.painstresscenter.com

Find Out How GABA . . .

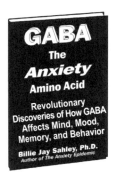

✔ Controls the anxiety "stop switch" in the brain

✔ Promotes smooth function of the gut and the brain together

✔ Works as a natural muscle relaxant

✔ Creates neurotransmitters needed for enhanced brain function

✔ Helps you think better and feel better naturally

The Healing Powers of Green Tea

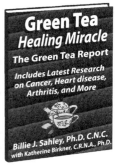

The healing properties of Green Tea offer a promise of healing that no other supplement can.

The properties of Green Tea EGCGs protect the body from dreaded diseases.

Until you see the research and read the results in this book, you can't begin to imagine the potential life saving properties of Green Tea.

Nature's Sleep Aid....Melatonin

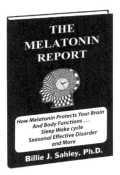

Melatonin is a neurohormone and antioxidant produced by the pineal gland located at the base of the brain.

Melatonin plays a part in producing critical neurotransmitters, hormones, brain function, and aging.

This report discusses the importance of Melatonin for the body, influencing Seasonal Affective Disorder (SAD), recovery from jet lag, normal sleep patterns, and the natural process of aging.

The Power of Amino Acids . . .

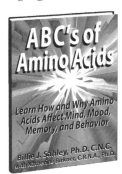

ABC's of Amino Acids explains the fundamentals in simple English.

Discover the step-by-step process of what happens in the brain.

Learn why these brain nutrients are essential to your health and ability to cope effectively.

To Order Call 1-800-669-2256 or go to www.painstresscenter.com

Relax with Theanine

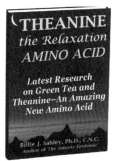

The amazing amino acid Theanine can change your life by helping you relax naturally without drowsiness or fear of addiction.

✓ *Diminishes symptoms of PMS, depression, and irritability*
✓ *Enhances memory and concentration*
✓ *Is superior to St. John's Wort, Kava Kava, and Valerian*
✓ *Lowers blood pressure and protects the heart*
✓ *Inhibits the growth of certain tumor (cancerous) cells*
✓ *Enhances your immune system and lowers anxiety and stress*

Millions of children and adults in the U.S. suffer from ADD or ADHD!

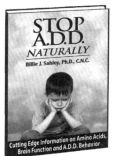

The orthomolecular program has been successfully used at the Pain & Stress Center to help hundreds of children whose symptoms range from mild to severe.

Correct brain deficiencies and imbalances *without drugs and without side effects!*

A complete guide for parents outling a total orthomolecular (drug-free) approach for positive, long-lasting results!

Natural Answers For Healing and Recovery

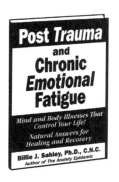

Chronic Emotional Fatigue (CEF) can control your mind and body. Millions of people live their lives in fear, anxiety, and pain. They go from doctor to doctor, but do not get the answers they are seeking.

CEF is not a drug deficiency, but a multitude of mental and physiological deficiencies that can be corrected naturally.

This book gives you a complete treatment plan for *natural healing and recovery—without drugs.*

Audio CDs from Pain & Stress Publications

To Order Call 1-800-669-2256 or go to www.painstresscenter.com

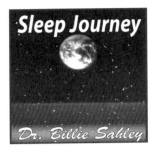
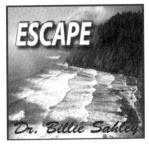
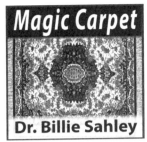
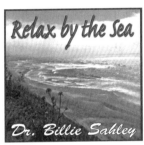
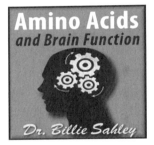
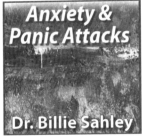
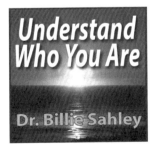
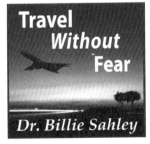
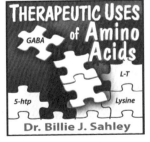
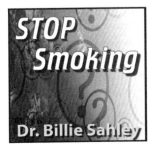
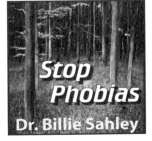
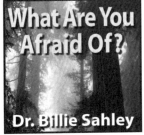

To Order Call 1-800-669-2256 or go to www.painstresscenter.com

More CD titles

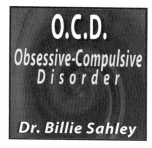
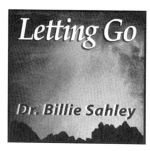
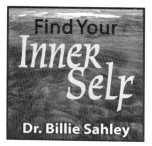
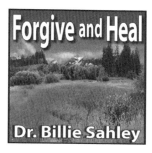
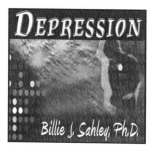
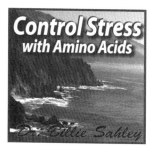
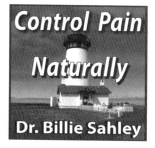
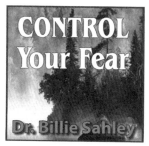
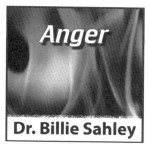
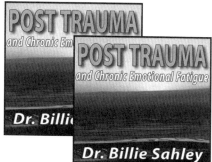

(Audio Book 2 Cd set)

About The Authors

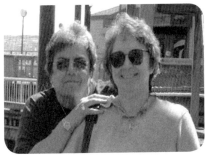

Billie J. Sahley, Ph.D., was founder and Executive Director of the Pain & Stress Center in San Antonio, now Helotes, Texas until 2011. She was a Board Certified Medical Psychotherapist & Psychodiagnostician, Behavior Therapist, Board Certified Expert in Traumatic Stress, Orthomolecular Therapist, and a Certified Nutritional Consultant. She was a Diplomate in the American Academy of Pain Management. Dr. Sahley was a graduate of the University of Texas, Clayton University School of Behavioral Medicine, and U.C.L.A. School of Integral Medicine. Additionally, she studied advanced nutritional biochemistry through Jeffrey Bland, Ph.D., at Institute of Functional Medicine. She was a member of the Huxley Foundation/Academy of Orthomolecular Medicine, Academy of Psychosomatic Medicine, North American Nutrition and Preventive Medicine Association, American Counseling Association, and American Academy of Pain Management. In addition, she held memberships in the Sports Medicine Foundation, American Association of Hypnotherapists, and American Mental Health Counselors Association.

Dr. Sahley wrote: ***The Anxiety Epidemic; GABA, The Anxiety Amino Acid; Post Trauma and Chronic Emotional Fatigue; A Natural Approach to Fibromyalgia and Chronic Pain; The Melatonin Report; Is Ritalin Necessary? The Ritalin Report; Stop A.D.D. Naturally; Theanine, The Relaxation Amino Acid; ABC's of Amino Acids;*** and has recorded numerous health and relaxation cds. She coauthored ***Break Your Prescribed Addiction, Green Tea Healing Miracle,*** and ***Control Alcoholism with Amino Acids and Nutrients.***

In addition, Dr. Sahley holds three U.S. patents for: SAF, Calms Kids (SAF For Kids), and Anxiety Control 24. Dr. Sahley devoted the majority of her time to research, writing, and development of natural products to address brain deficiencies.

Kathy Birkner is Director and a C.R.N.A., Pain Therapist at the Pain & Stress Center in Helotes, TX. She is a Registered Nurse, Certified Registered Nurse Anesthetist, Advanced Nurse Practitioner, Orthomolecular Therapist, and a Certified Nutritional Consultant. She is a Diplomate in the American Academy of Pain Management. She attended Brackenridge Hospital School of Nursing, University of Texas at Austin, Southwest Missouri School of Anesthesia, Southwest Missouri State University, and Clayton University. She holds degrees in nursing, nutrition, and behavior therapy. Dr. Birkner has done graduate studies through the Center for Integral Medicine and U.C.L.A. Medical School, under the direction of Dr. David Bresler. Additionally, she has studied advanced nutritional biochemistry through Jeffrey Bland, Ph.D., at Institute of Functional Medicine. She is a member of the American Association of Nurse Anesthetists, Texas Association of Nurse Anesthetists and American Academy of Pain Management. She is author of ***Breaking Your Sugar Habit Cookbook*** and coauthored ***Break Your Prescribed Addiction, Green Tea Healing Miracle,*** and ***Control Alcoholism with Amino Acids and Nutrients.***

Even though Dr. Sahley has passed, her dream and work lives on. In the spirit of Dr. Sahley's research and innovation, Dr. Birkner continues to do research into alternatives at Pain & Stress Center offering people hope and wellness. Dr. Birkner has updated this book to keep the information current and relative.